THE FIRST-TIME MOM'S PREGNANCY JOURNAL

Copyright © 2019 by Rockridge Press, Emeryville, California

No part of this publication may be reproduced, stored in a retrieval system or transmitted in any form or by any means, electronic, mechanical, photocopying, recording, scanning or otherwise, except as permitted under Sections 107 or 108 of the 1976 United States Copyright Act, without the prior written permission of the Publisher. Requests to the Publisher for permission should be addressed to the Permissions Department, Rockridge Press, 6005 Shellmound Street, Suite 175, Emeryville, CA 94608.

Limit of Liability/Disclaimer of Warranty: The Publisher and the author make no representations or warranties with respect to the accuracy or completeness of the contents of this work and specifically disclaim all warranties, including without limitation warranties of fitness for a particular purpose. No warranty may be created or extended by sales or promotional materials. The advice and strategies contained herein may not be suitable for every situation. This work is sold with the understanding that the Publisher is not engaged in rendering medical, legal, or other professional advice or services. If professional assistance is required, the services of a competent professional person should be sought. Neither the Publisher nor the author shall be liable for damages arising herefrom. The fact that an individual, organization or website is referred to in this work as a citation and/or potential source of further information does not mean that the author or the Publisher endorses the information the individual, organization or website may provide or recommendations they/it may make. Further, readers should be aware that Internet websites listed in this work may have changed or disappeared between when this work was written and when it is read.

For general information on our other products and services or to obtain technical support, please contact our Customer Care Department within the U.S. at (866) 744-2665, or outside the U.S. at (510) 253-0500.

Rockridge Press publishes its books in a variety of electronic and print formats. Some content that appears in print may not be available in electronic books, and vice versa.

TRADEMARKS: Rockridge Press and the Rockridge Press logo are trademarks or registered trademarks of Callisto Media Inc. and/or its affiliates, in the United States and other countries, and may not be used without written permission. All other trademarks are the property of their respective owners. Rockridge Press is not associated with any product or vendor mentioned in this book.

Interior and Cover Designer: Lisa Forde
Art Manager: Sara Feinstein
Editor: Kim Suarez

Production Editor: Ashley Polikoff
Illustrations: Frances MacLeod

ISBN: 978-1-64152-450-6

This Journal Belongs to

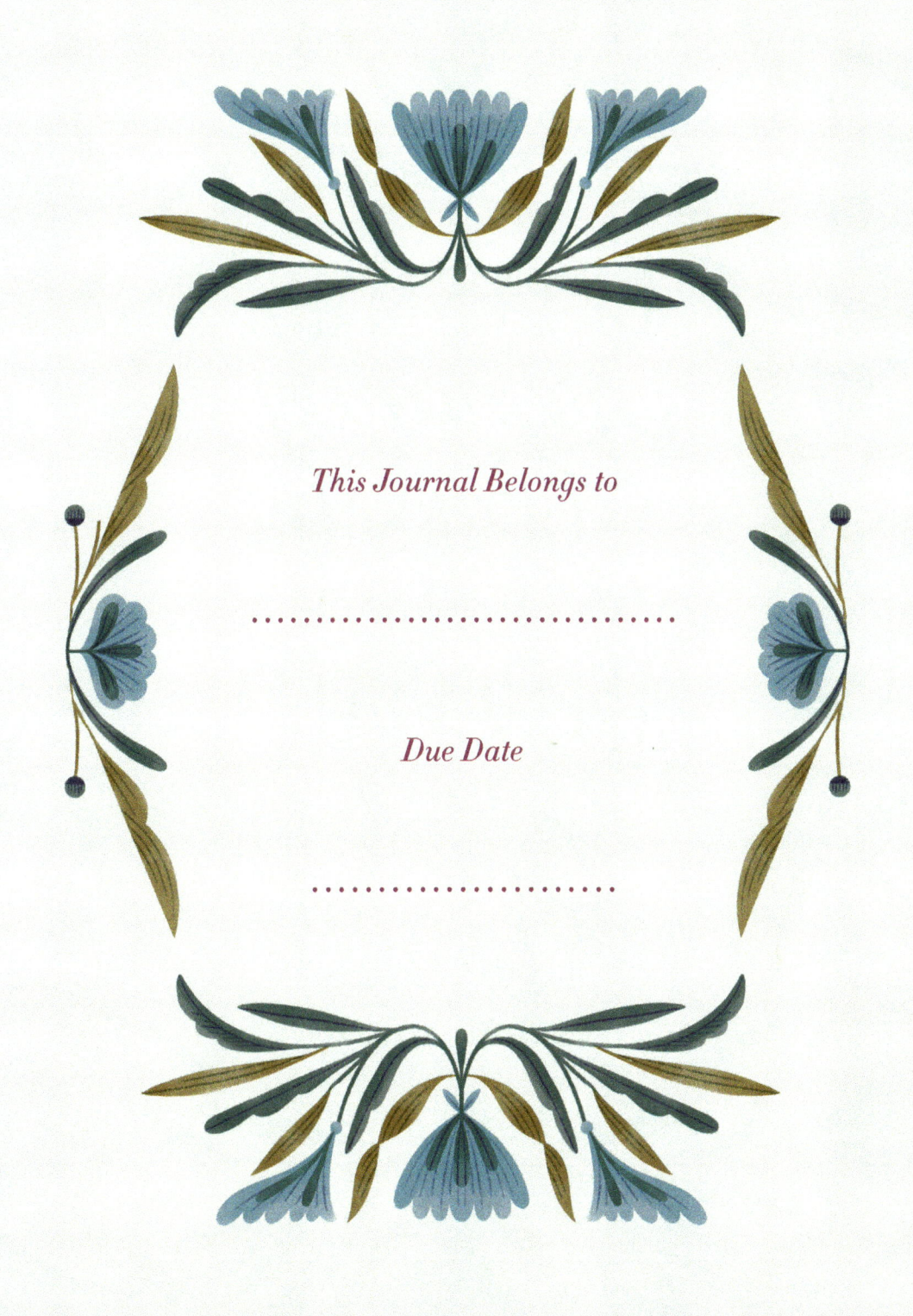

....

Due Date

....

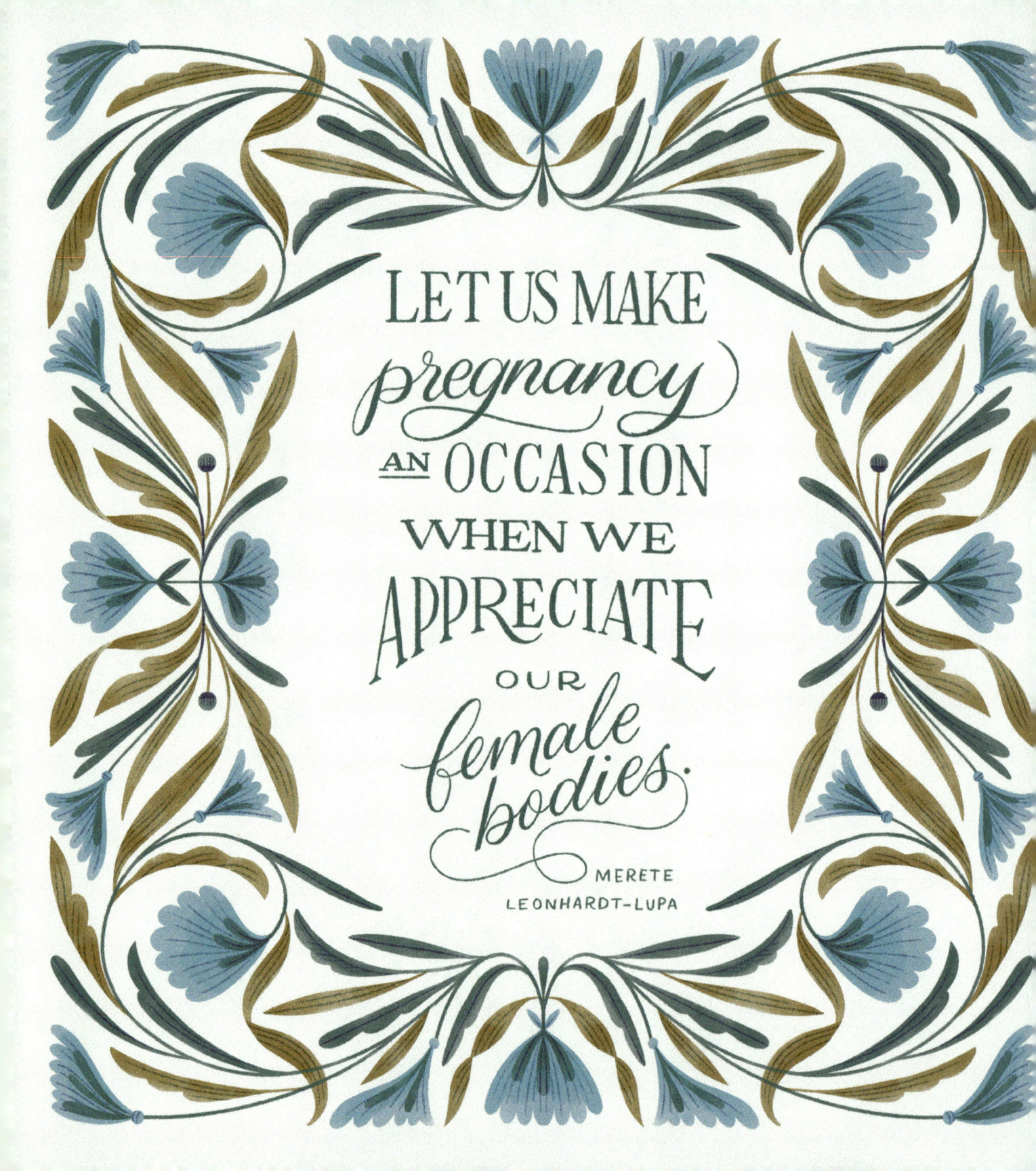

Let us make *pregnancy* an occasion when we appreciate our *female bodies.*

—Merete Leonhardt-Lupa

The
First-Time Mom's
Pregnancy
Journal

Monthly Checklists, Activities & Journal Prompts

Aubrey Grossen

Illustrations by Frances MacLeod

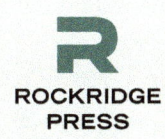

ROCKRIDGE PRESS

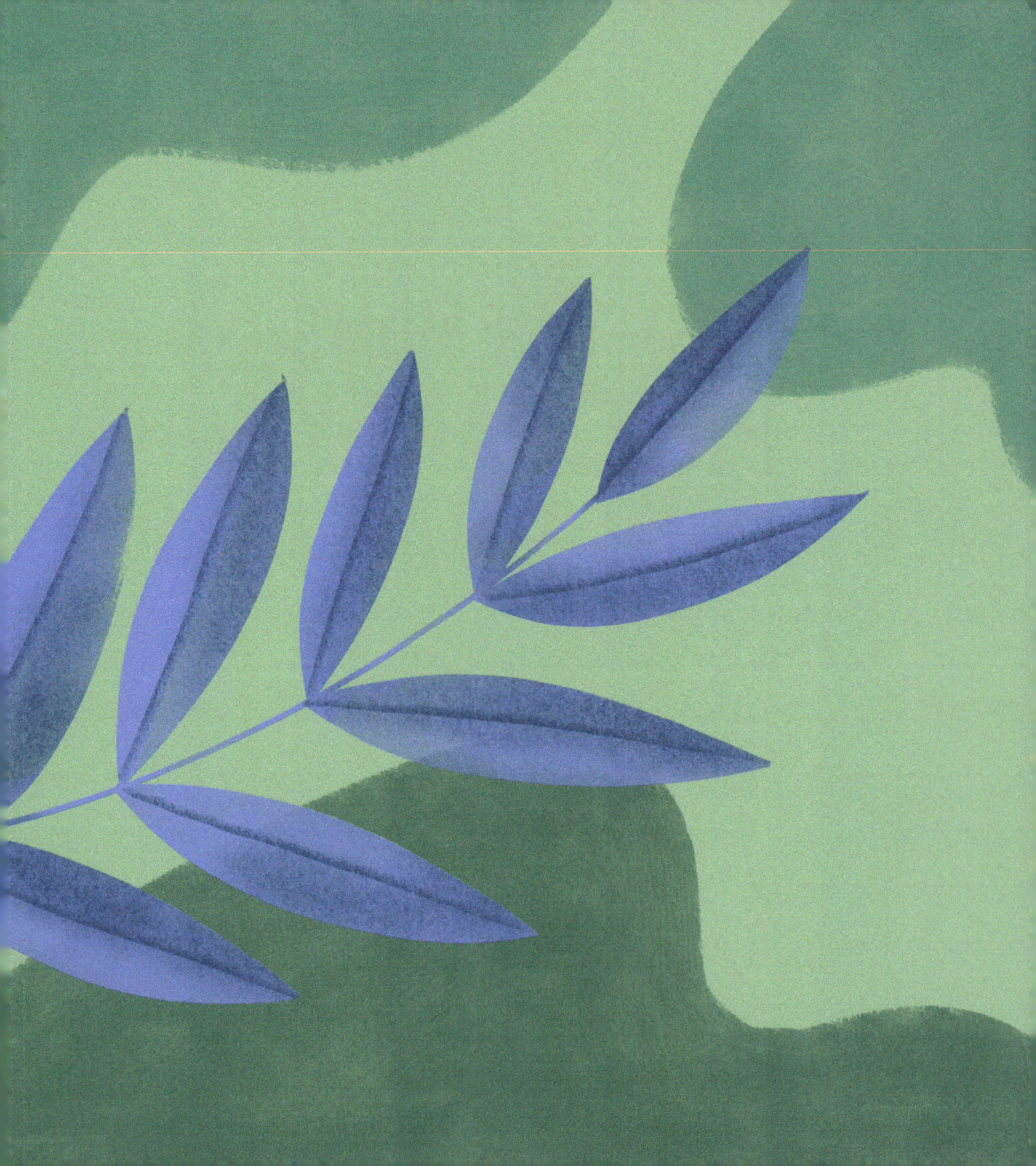

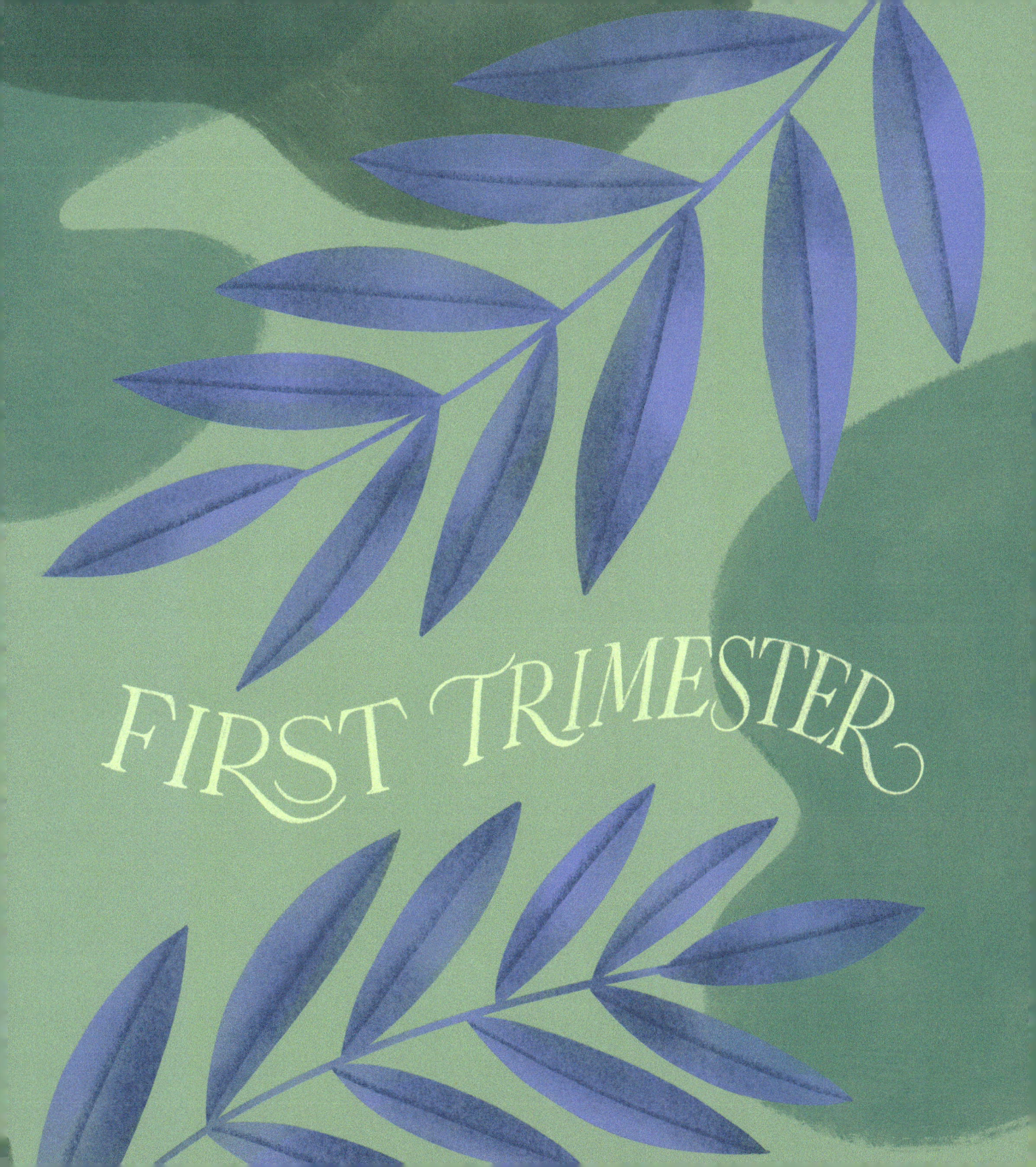

FIRST TRIMESTER

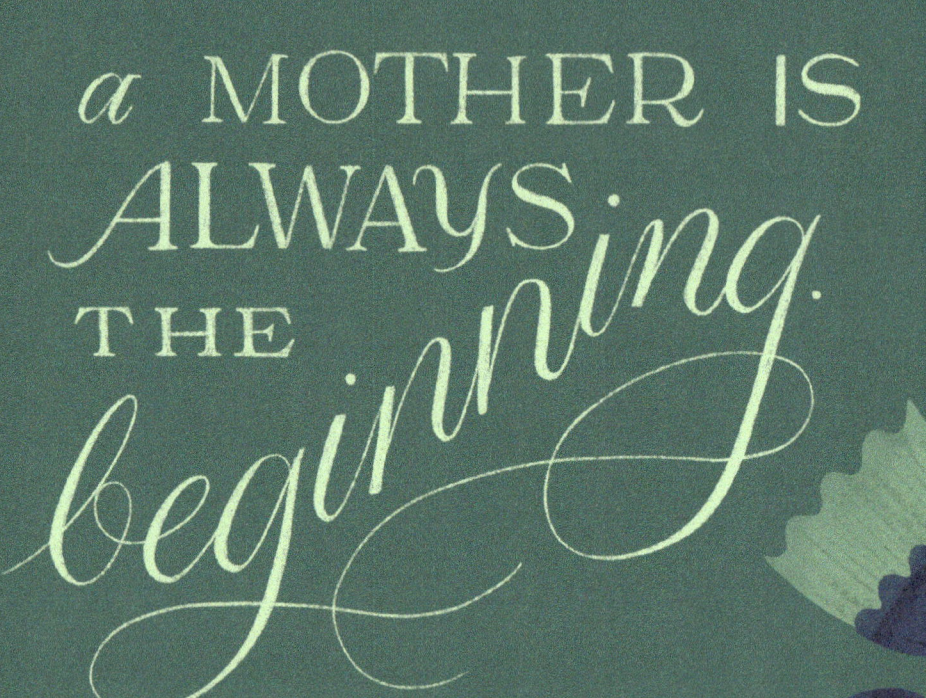

A MOTHER IS ALWAYS THE *beginning*. SHE IS HOW THINGS BEGIN.

AMY TAN, *THE BONESETTER'S DAUGHTER*

FIRST-TRIMESTER ULTRASOUND

PHOTO HERE

I'M PREGNANT!

When and where I found out _____

_____

My reaction _____

_____

Who I told first _____

_____

Their reaction _____

_____

MONTH 1: FIRST-TIME MOM'S FIRSTS

First sign or symptom of pregnancy _____

_____

First cry caused by hormones _____

_____

First unusual craving _____

_____

WEEKS 1 TO 4

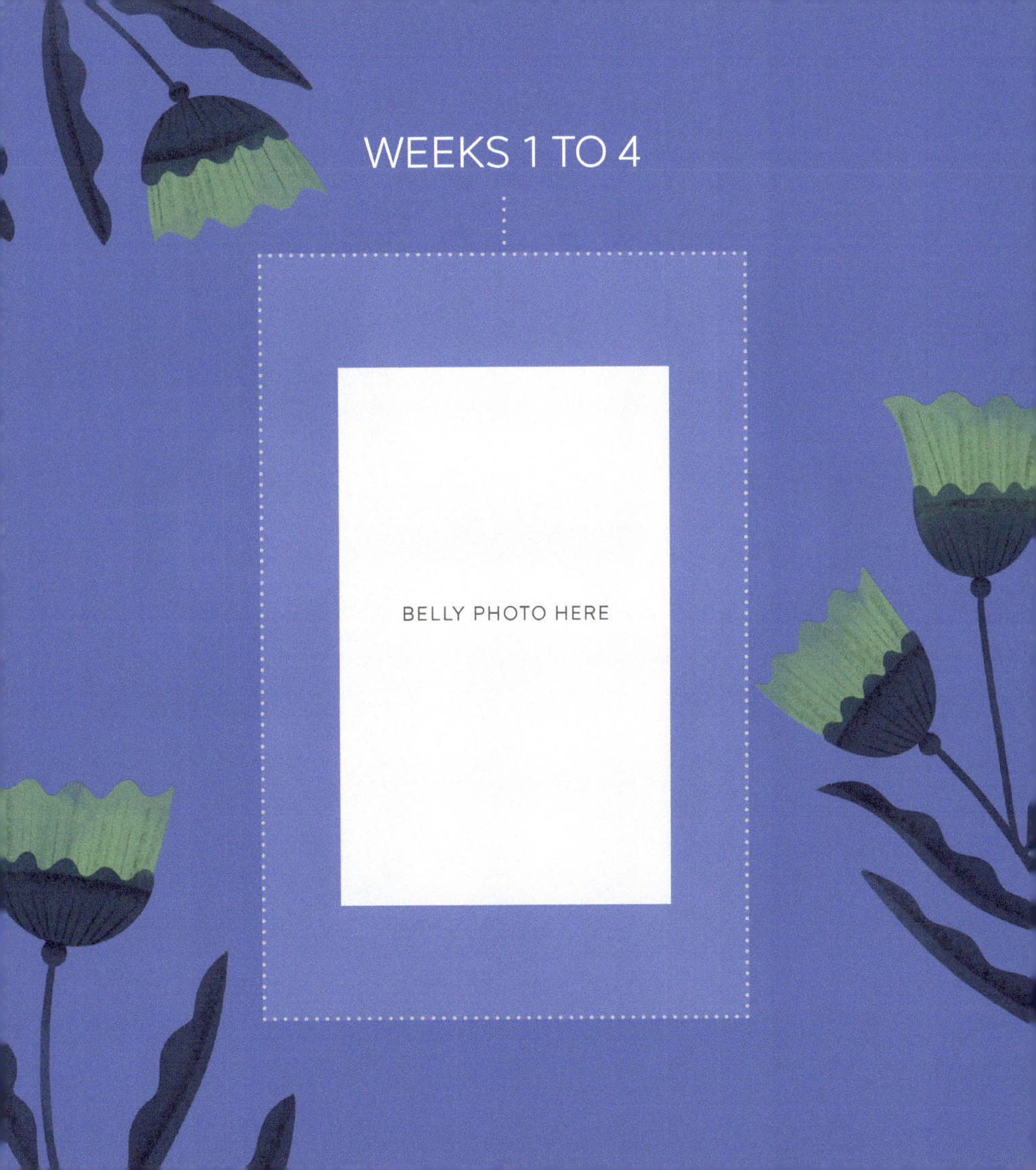

BELLY PHOTO HERE

SIZE COMPARISON

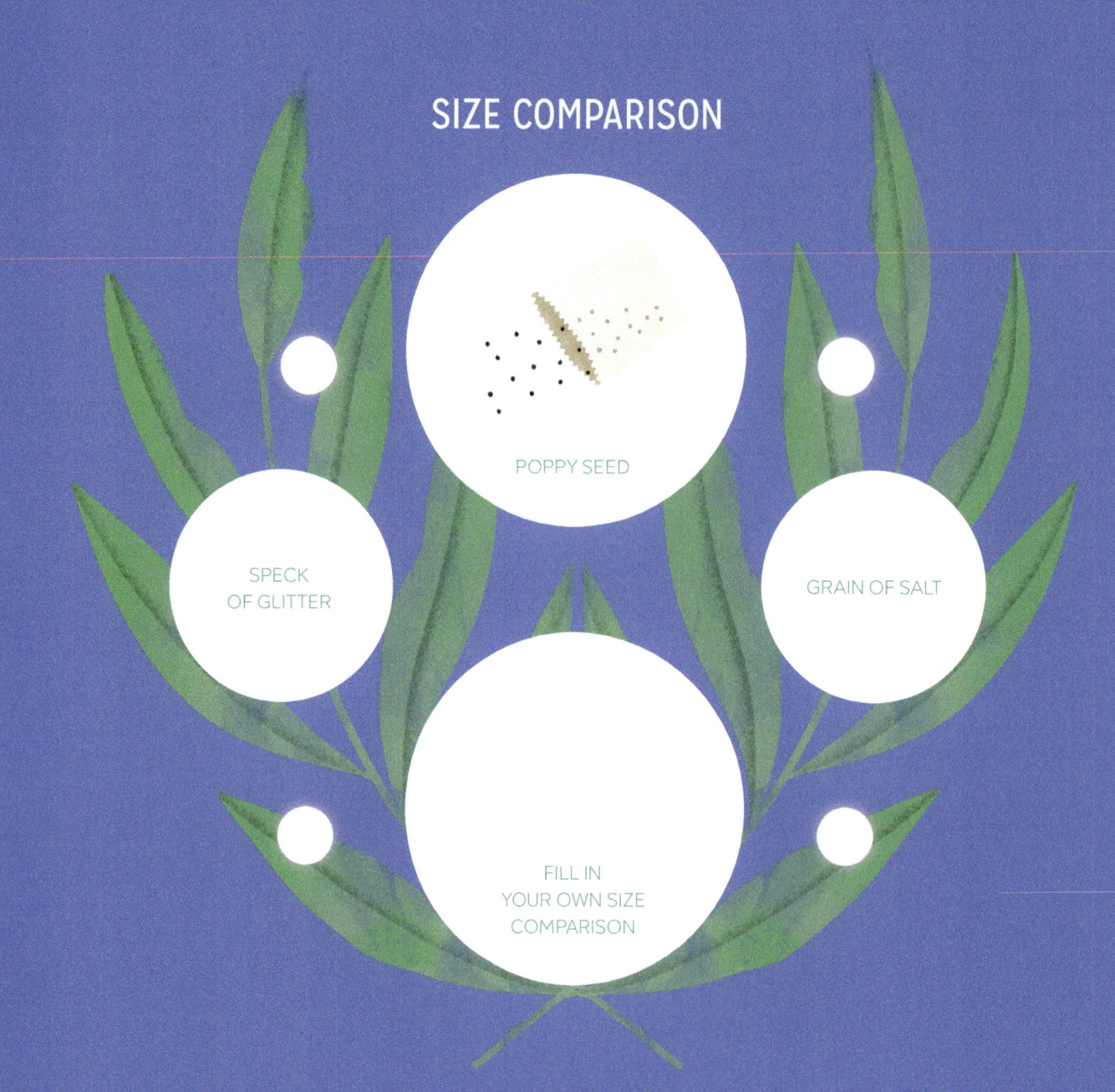

POPPY SEED

SPECK OF GLITTER

GRAIN OF SALT

FILL IN YOUR OWN SIZE COMPARISON

By the end of this month, your baby is about 2 millimeters long.

PREGNANCY STATS TRACKER

Body

What are your feelings toward your new pregnant body? _____

_____

Some women feel cramping or have a little bit of bleeding in the beginning of pregnancy, when the egg attaches to the uterine wall. Have you felt or experienced these or any other unpleasant symptoms? _____

_____

_____

Have you noticed any changes in your breasts this month? _____

_____

_____

Baby

Your baby's face is starting to form. Blood cells are taking shape, and circulation is beginning. In addition, your placenta—a round, flat organ that transfers nutrients from you to your baby—has developed. It's amazing to think that all of this growth happens to something as small as the period at the end of this sentence. How does it feel to realize that all of this is happening in your body? _____

_____

_____

Are you giving up any foods or habits to keep your baby healthy? _____

_____

_____

PRENATAL APPOINTMENTS

DATE	WEEK	WEIGHT	TESTS CONDUCTED	QUESTIONS FOR DOCTOR/MIDWIFE

MONTH 1 CHECKLIST

Home

- Designate a room or spot in your home where you can collect baby-related items.
- Decide where your baby will sleep. Will they spend the first six months in your bedroom? In a separate room?
- Declutter as much as you can to make space for the baby's items, but keep in mind that babies don't need as much as you think they do.
- _____
- _____
- _____

Self-Care

- Get some rest. Your body is working hard to help your baby develop.
- Start taking prenatal vitamins, supplements, or any other medications recommended by your doctor/midwife.
- If you are starting to have bouts of nausea in the morning or throughout your day, keep a stash of Gatorade, ginger tablets or cookies, Preggie Pops, and peppermint gum or lip balm handy to help you survive the hard stretches. Also try to sleep through the worst part, if your schedule allows.
- Watch your favorite movie or the comedy *Baby Mama* to get you amped up or just for a good laugh—and maybe even a good cry!
- _____
- _____
- _____

Baby

- Use an online due-date calculator to figure out your due date. Remember that this date is just a rough estimate. When you go to your first prenatal appointment, your doctor/midwife should give you a better idea of your due date based on your last period and an ultrasound. This date is subject to change as your pregnancy continues.

- Sign up to receive updates on your baby's development from BabyCenter.com or a similar website. Or download a development-tracking app such as BabyCenter, the Bump, Ovia, Glow Nurture, and What to Expect.

- Start thinking about baby names.

- Think about what kind of delivery you want to have. Medicated? Unmedicated?

- Start researching baby books and parenting books to find a few you would like to read.

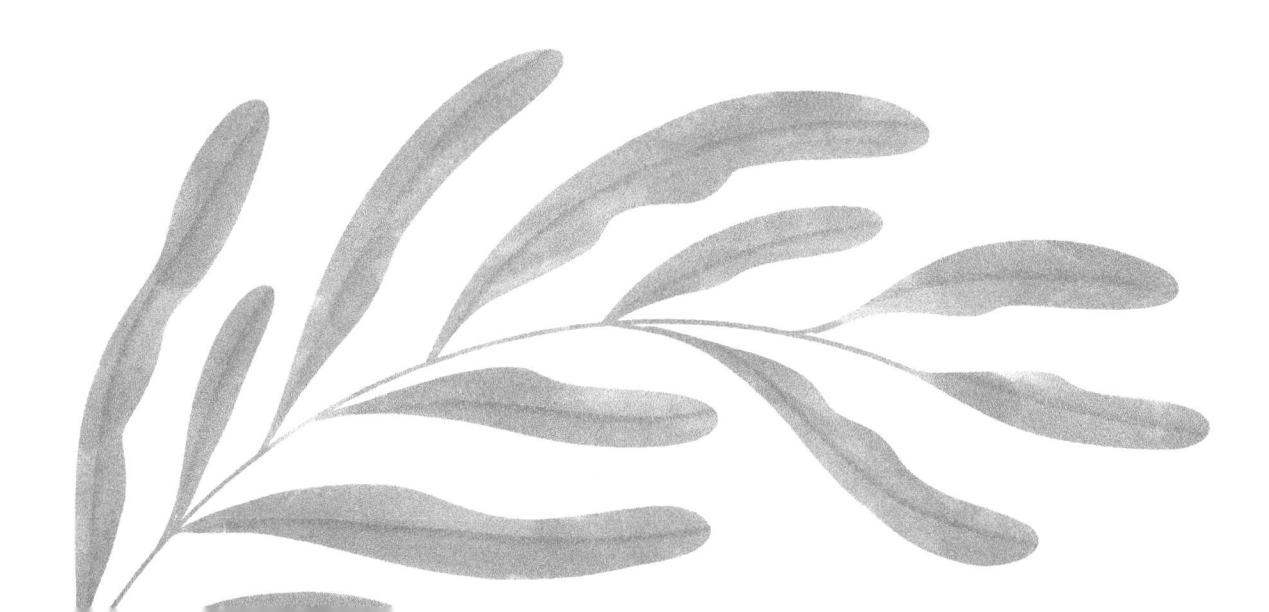

- _____
- _____
- _____

Medical

- Find a good doctor/midwife by asking close friends and family. You'll want one who is right for you and your personality. Do you prefer someone who gets right to the point? More talkative and friendly? Do you have a gender preference? Reading reviews online or asking members of a Facebook group, such as the Mamahood Blog community (themamahoodblog.com), can also help you find a good one.

- Schedule your first prenatal appointment with your doctor/midwife. One thing to ask at that appointment is whether they can deliver your baby at the hospital you're hoping for. If you have health insurance, you'll need to know if it will cover delivery at that hospital.

- Call your health insurance provider to discuss what you need to know regarding pregnancy-related medical expenses.

- Make a list of questions to ask and topics to discuss with your doctor/midwife at every visit. Keep this list on your phone so that you don't forget to take it to your appointments. For example, any different symptoms you've been feeling, questions about prenatal vitamins, the food you're eating, or any other questions you might have. (Pregnancy brain is real!)

- _____
- _____
- _____

Important Events

- Start thinking about your long-term plans for when the baby comes.
- Figure out when you will tell your close family and friends about your pregnancy. This is a personal choice, but one advantage of telling those closest to you is having their support if you need it.
- Calculate when you'll be able to find out your baby's gender. It can usually be seen on an ultrasound around the 20-week mark. If you want to know sooner, you can ask your doctor/midwife for a blood test that can detect the gender.
- _____
- _____
- _____

DAILY REMINDERS

- Drink 10 cups of water over the course of the day.
- Take your prenatal vitamin.
- Eat at least three meals and three snacks.

Activity #1

Start to daydream about your nursery! Write down some ideas and/or use actual color swatches and pictures to show what you want in your nursery.

Activity #2

Write a brief letter to your baby discussing how you feel about being pregnant and describing what your life looks like right now.

Activity #3

Start thinking of potential baby names. You can use this table to list the girls' and boys' names you like.

BOYS' NAMES	GIRLS' NAMES

Activity #4

Daydream about your baby. What is their personality like? Will they be like you? What do they look like? Either draw an image or use words to describe your thoughts.

Gratitude

What do you feel especially grateful for during this first month of your pregnancy?

_____
_____
_____
_____
_____
_____

Challenge

What has been the hardest part physically? Emotionally?

_____
_____
_____
_____
_____
_____

Reflection

How do those closest to you feel about what's going on now that you're pregnant?

_____
_____
_____
_____
_____

Observation

What is the biggest change your body has gone through these past few weeks?

_____
_____
_____
_____
_____

FREESTYLE JOURNAL

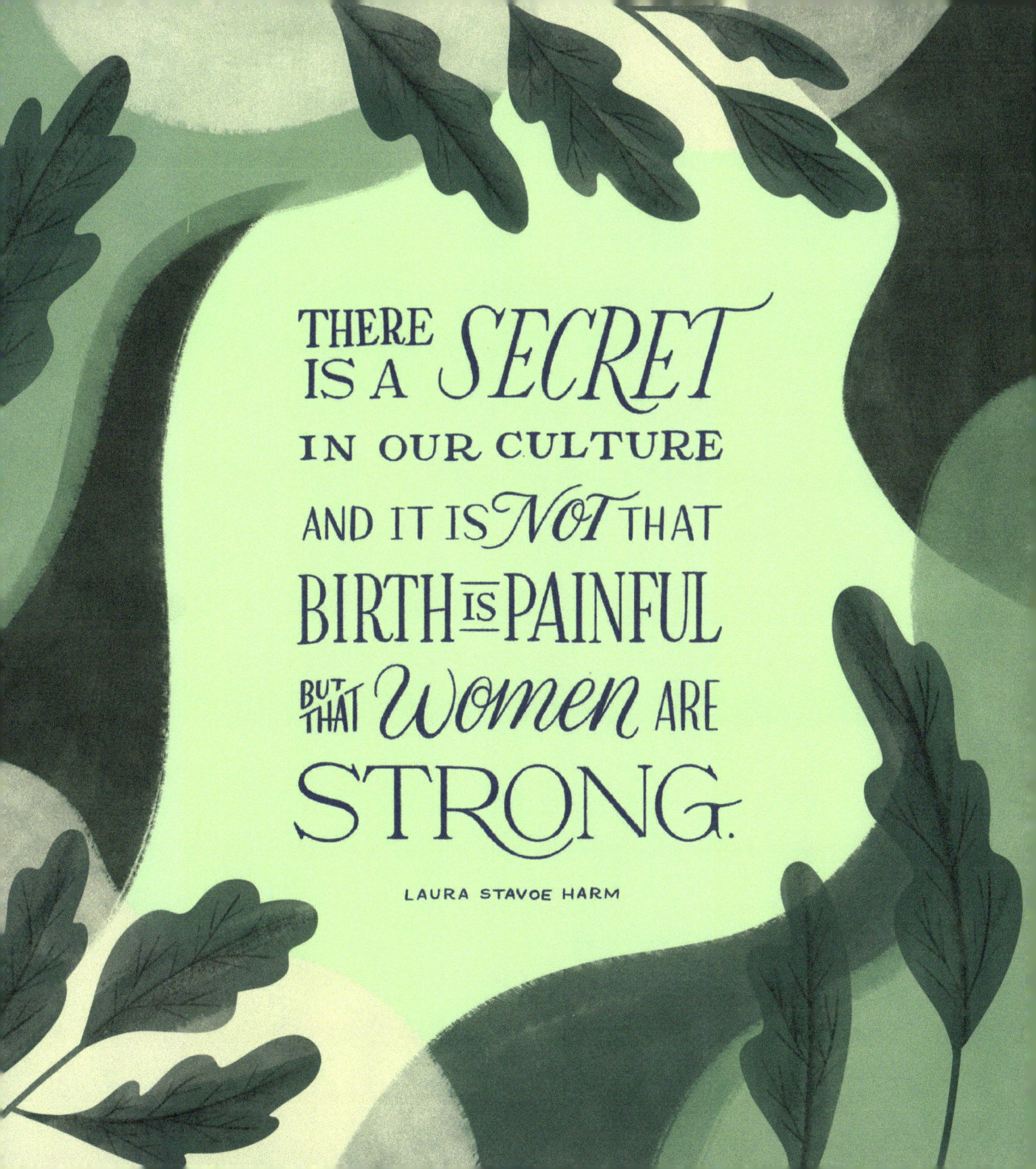

THERE IS A *SECRET* IN OUR CULTURE AND IT IS *NOT* THAT BIRTH IS PAINFUL BUT THAT *WOMEN* ARE STRONG.

— LAURA STAVOE HARM

MONTH 2: FIRST-TIME MOM'S FIRSTS

First time hearing your baby's heartbeat _____
_____
_____
_____

First impressions of your doctor/midwife _____
_____
_____
_____

First day feeling morning sickness _____
_____
_____
_____

First body changes you've noticed _____
_____
_____
_____

First time you've felt like eating something you normally wouldn't eat _____
_____
_____
_____

WEEKS 5 TO 8

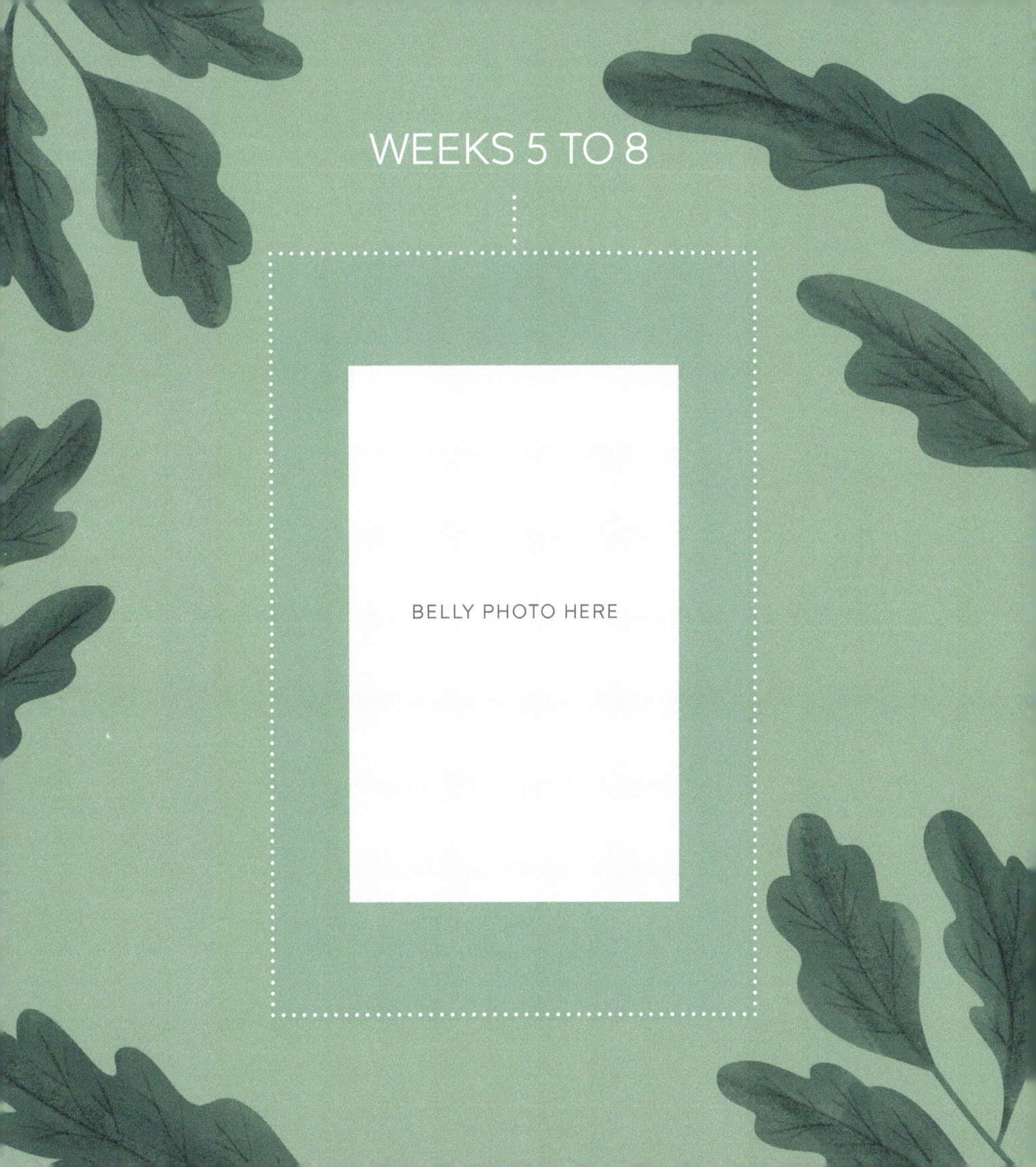

BELLY PHOTO HERE

SIZE COMPARISON

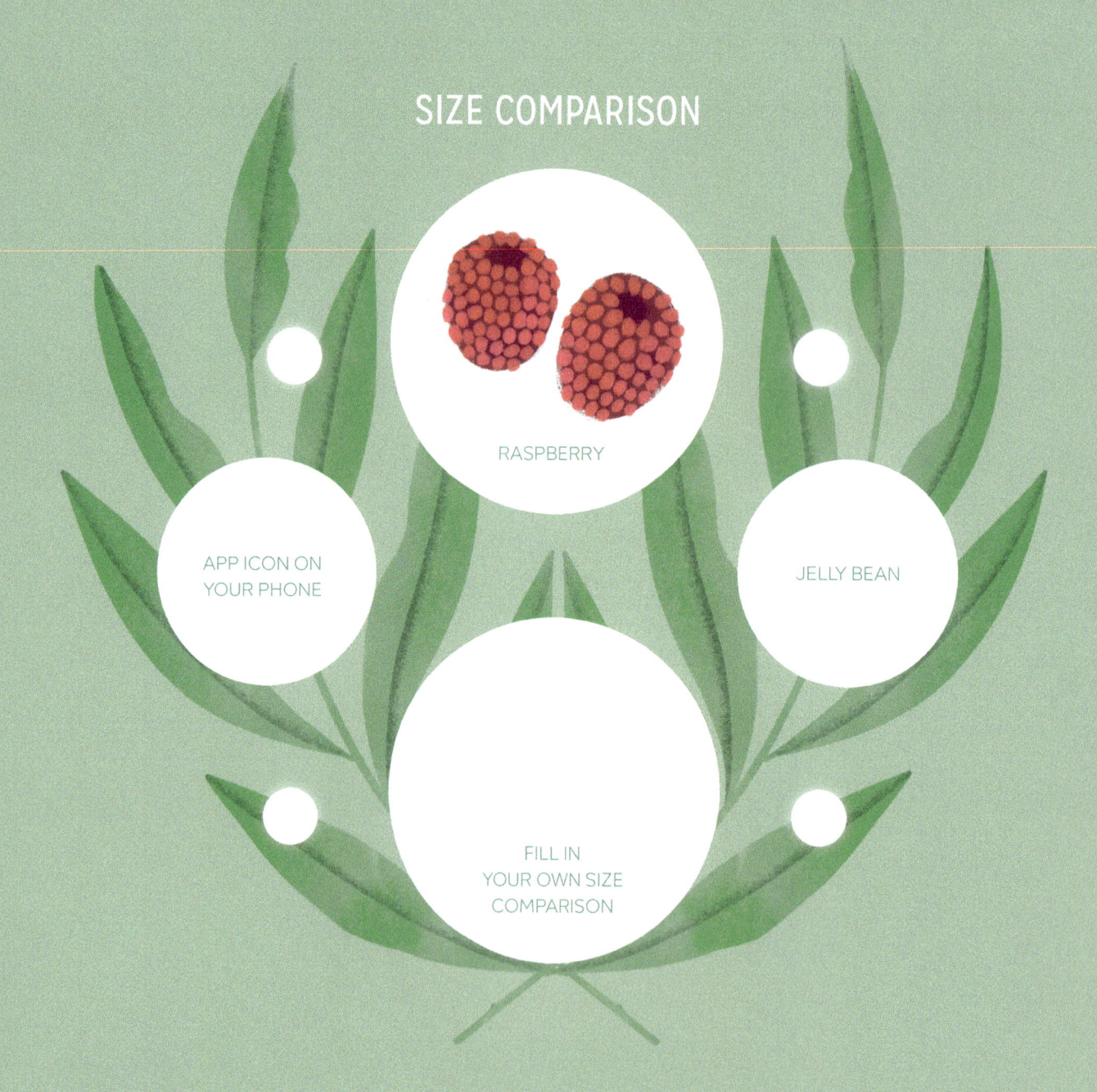

RASPBERRY

APP ICON ON YOUR PHONE

JELLY BEAN

FILL IN YOUR OWN SIZE COMPARISON

By the end of this month, your baby is about 1 inch long and weighs about one-third of an ounce; your baby's head is about one-third of their body size.

PREGNANCY STATS TRACKER

Body

Have you had any breast tenderness? _____
_____
_____

Are you and the bathroom becoming good friends yet? Frequent urination is common during pregnancy. _____
_____
_____

Do you have morning sickness? Does it affect you throughout the day or only part of the day?
_____
_____

Baby

What updates did the doctor/midwife give you about your baby at your first prenatal appointment? _____
_____

Have you noticed any feelings for or emotional connection to your baby? Some people don't feel anything until they give birth. So if you don't right now, that's okay. _____
_____
_____

What have you found interesting about the development of your baby so far in your pregnancy?
_____
_____
_____

PRENATAL APPOINTMENTS

DATE	WEEK	WEIGHT	TESTS CONDUCTED	QUESTIONS FOR DOCTOR/MIDWIFE

MONTH 2 CHECKLIST

Home

- Envision what your new routine will be when the baby comes.
- Research the latest baby products, and, if you need them, figure out where you will put them in your home.
- Decide if you would like a doula (a birth coach) to help you before, during, and/or after birth.
- _____
- _____
- _____

Self-Care

- Go easy on yourself if you can't do everything right now.
- Allow yourself to feel sad or frustrated for feeling like pregnancy is hard.
- Confide in a trusted friend about the good and the bad of pregnancy.
- Take a warm bath (not too hot) and eat snacks while you bathe. (Trust me on this one; it's a luxury!)
- Because you're more than likely feeling fatigued, ask others to help around the house or enlist the help of a friend.

- _____
- _____
- _____

Baby

- Go to a baby store and try out the strollers. Believe me when I say that stroller shopping is just about as intense as car shopping. There are so many different bells and whistles. There are guides online offering different reviews to help you figure out your preferences. Remember to consider how you will store the stroller when you're not using it.
- Start to narrow down names to the ones you like best.
- Talk to friends who have given birth to learn what their preferences were during their deliveries. Decide what details are important to you.
- _____
- _____
- _____

Medical

- Schedule your next few appointments with your doctor/midwife.
- Call your doctor/midwife if you have any questions or concerns. It's better to double-check than to sit at home and worry.
- Make sure you have confidence in your doctor/midwife and are on board with their

recommendations. If anything feels off, try to resolve the issue, or find a new doctor/midwife before your second trimester. You can always change at any point in your pregnancy, but it's easier to stay with the same person the whole time.

- Watch for any spotting or cramping, and call your doctor/midwife right away if something doesn't feel right.

- _____
- _____
- _____

Important Events

- Think of ways you'd like to announce your pregnancy to the special people in your life.

- _____
- _____
- _____

DAILY REMINDERS

○ Drink 10 cups of water over the course of the day.

○ Take your prenatal vitamin.

○ Eat at least three meals and three snacks.

Activity #1

In the following table, list the things you are most excited about in becoming a mom and things you are least excited about.

MOST EXCITED ABOUT	LEAST EXCITED ABOUT

Activity #2

On the left side of the timetable, write down your current daily schedule by the hour. On the other side, write down what you think your daily schedule will look like when the baby comes.

MY CURRENT DAILY SCHEDULE	MY SCHEDULE AFTER THE BABY

Activity #3

Make a list of the foods you loved before you got pregnant but can't stand now to see how your palate has changed since you became pregnant.

_____

_____

_____

_____

_____

_____

Activity #4

Are you loving pregnancy so far? Yes or no?

Write down what you love or hate about it.

LOVE IT	HATE IT

Gratitude

Who are you most excited to share your pregnancy news with and why?

_____
_____
_____
_____
_____
_____
_____

Challenge

If you have pregnancy fatigue or any other symptoms, how are you dealing with them?

_____
_____
_____
_____
_____
_____

Reflection

What kind of parent do you think you'll be?

_____
_____
_____
_____
_____
_____
_____

Observation

What's the weirdest thing your body has done so far?

_____
_____
_____
_____
_____
_____

FREESTYLE JOURNAL

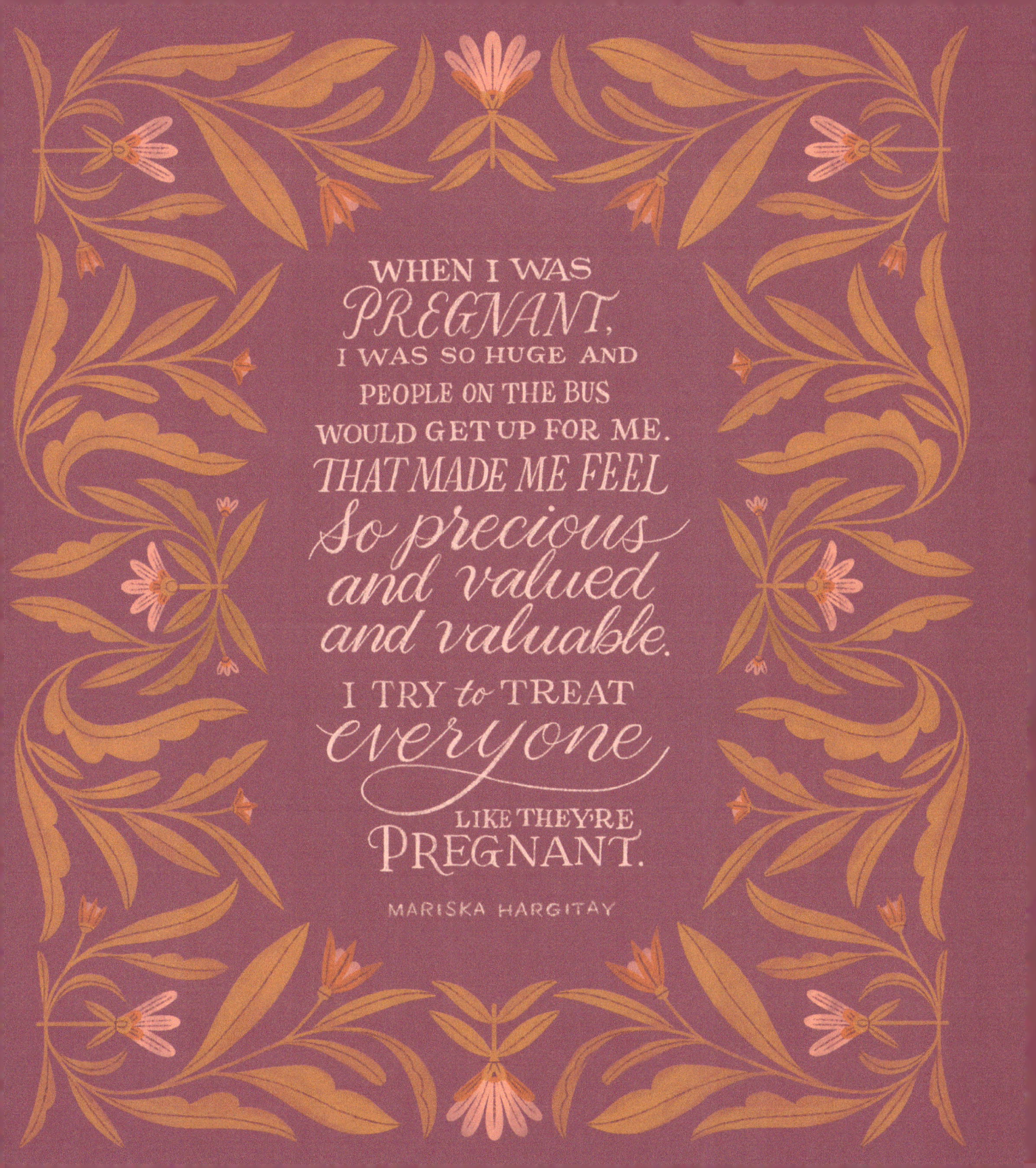

WHEN I WAS PREGNANT, I WAS SO HUGE AND PEOPLE ON THE BUS WOULD GET UP FOR ME. THAT MADE ME FEEL *so precious and valued and valuable.* I TRY *to* TREAT *everyone* LIKE THEY'RE PREGNANT.

— MARISKA HARGITAY

MONTH 3: FIRST-TIME MOM'S FIRSTS

First time you felt pregnant (not just like you had a "food baby")

First ultrasound appointment

First time you felt love for your baby

First pregnancy-related stress you've had

First time someone asked if you were pregnant

WEEKS 9 TO 12

BELLY PHOTO HERE

SIZE COMPARISON

PLUMS

SMALL CACTUS

PING-PONG BALL

FILL IN YOUR OWN SIZE COMPARISON

By the end of this month, your baby is
3 to 4 inches long and weighs about 1 ounce.

PREGNANCY STATS TRACKER

Body

How have you been feeling lately? Your moods might feel a little bit all over the place. _____
_____

What does morning sickness look like for you? _____
_____

How are you feeling stress-wise? _____
_____

How are you feeling fatigue-wise? _____
_____

Baby

Do you think you know your baby's gender? _____
_____

Some women can feel movements as early as 12 weeks; have you felt any? _____
_____

Was your baby measuring on schedule at your last prenatal appointment? _____
_____
_____

Have you had any health concerns so far? _____
_____
_____

PRENATAL APPOINTMENTS

DATE	WEEK	WEIGHT	TESTS CONDUCTED	QUESTIONS FOR DOCTOR/MIDWIFE

MONTH 3 CHECKLIST

Home

- When you have the energy, deep clean your home but without exposing yourself to chemicals. You could focus on the clutter while someone else wipes everything down, or you could hire a cleaning service.
- If you have a hard time asking for help, come up with a code word to say when you need extra help from someone close to you. That person could also help you ask other close friends and family for additional support.
- Don't lift heavy items.
- Buy a houseplant that you can watch grow while your baby grows.
- _____
- _____
- _____

Self-Care

- Make sure to eat protein-rich snacks throughout the day to combat the empty-pit stomachaches that are common during pregnancy.
- Go shopping for maternity clothes and/or borrow clothes from friends.

- Continue to take your prenatal vitamin and any other supplements your doctor/midwife recommends.
- Lotion up! It's common to experience dry skin during pregnancy, so make sure to moisturize.
- Treat yourself to a prenatal massage if your doctor/midwife approves.
- Have you had any back or neck problems? Get adjusted by a chiropractor if needed.
- _____
- _____
- _____

Baby

- Find other moms whose babies are due around the same time as yours. They could be part of your circle of friends or your family, or you could find them via social media. Even if you don't know them personally, it's fun to connect with other moms who are in your same boat.
- Choose your top two favorite baby names—one for a boy and one for a girl.
- Keep a stash of healthy snacks in your bag or car in case you get an empty-pit stomachache while you're out and about.
- _____
- _____
- _____

Medical

- Make sure to have your second prenatal appointment and any additional appointments your doctor/midwife recommends. Find out if you need any extra tests, and don't worry if you do.
- Decide if you want the nuchal translucency scan, which tests for Down syndrome or other chromosomal abnormalities.
- _____
- _____

Important Events

- If you've decided to learn your baby's gender before birth, think about whether you want to share it with others. If so, how do you want do it? A gender-reveal party? An email with a clever photo? Privately telling others one by one? Write down your own ideas.
- _____
- _____

DAILY REMINDERS

- Drink 10 cups of water over the course of the day.
- Take your prenatal vitamin.
- Eat at least three meals and three snacks.

Activity #1

Inside the circle below, write down all of your positive feelings toward pregnancy. Outside the circle, write down all your negative feelings toward pregnancy.

Try to focus on what's inside the circle.

Activity #2

Write down five things you love about your new pregnant body.
In what ways do you feel strong?

1. _____

2. _____

3. _____

4. _____

5. _____

Activity #3

Research gender-reveal ideas online and write down some of your favorites. If you are not having a gender-reveal event or do not wish to know the baby's gender, write about your decision below.

_____
_____
_____
_____
_____
_____
_____
_____
_____
_____

Activity #4

Close your eyes. Breathe in deeply and exhale deeply for one minute. Bring in positive thoughts as you inhale, and allow your shoulders to relax and your body to release stress as you exhale. Afterward, write down the positive thoughts.

_____
_____
_____
_____
_____
_____
_____
_____
_____
_____

Gratitude

What has brought you the most joy since you found out you were pregnant?

_____
_____
_____
_____
_____

Challenge

What pregnancy symptom has been the hardest for you during the first trimester?

_____
_____
_____
_____
_____

Reflection

Are there things that you'd like to keep private during your pregnancy? Why or why not?

_____
_____
_____
_____
_____

Observation

Do you hope to have a boy or a girl? Is it a strong preference?

_____
_____
_____
_____
_____

FREESTYLE JOURNAL

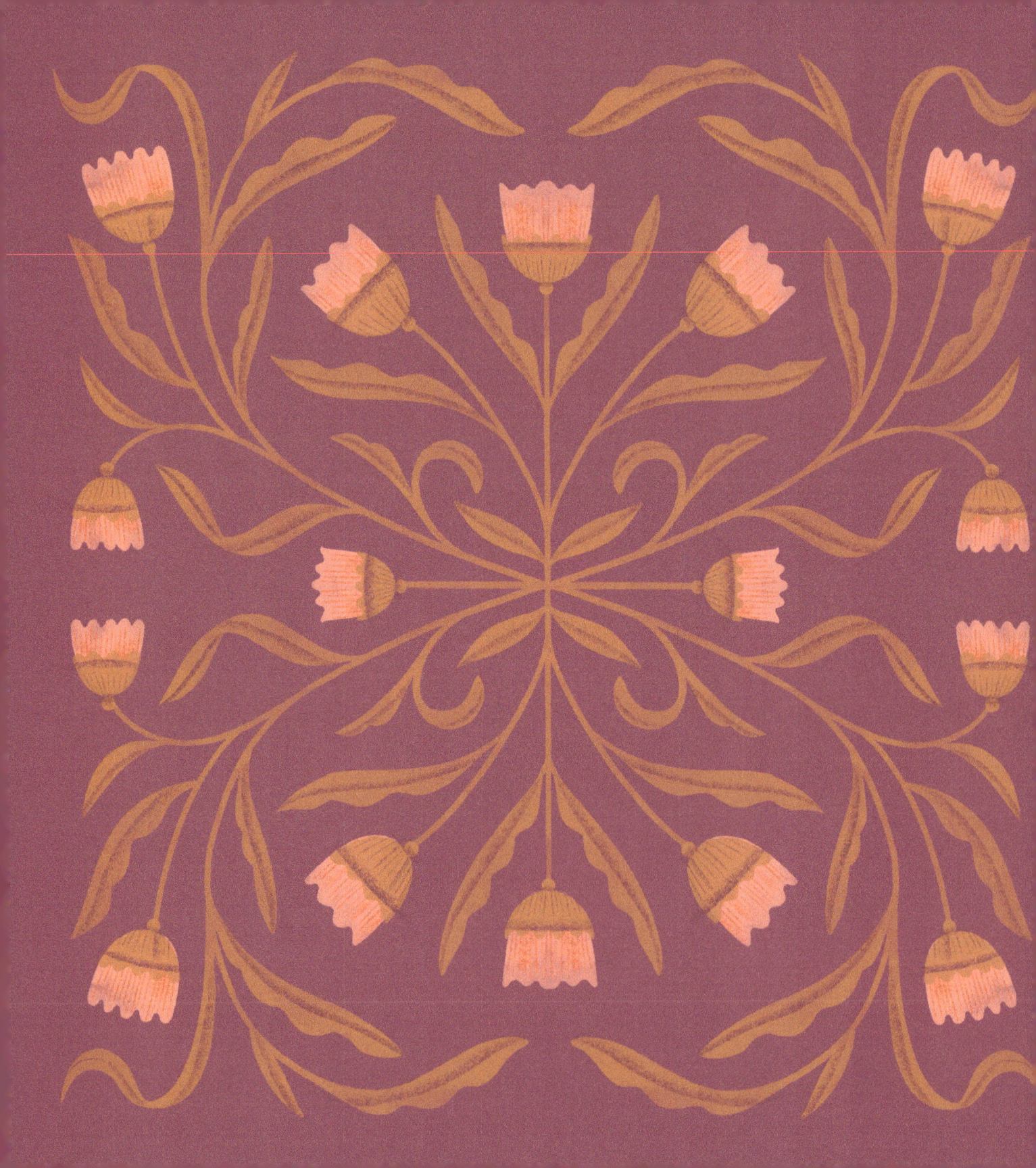

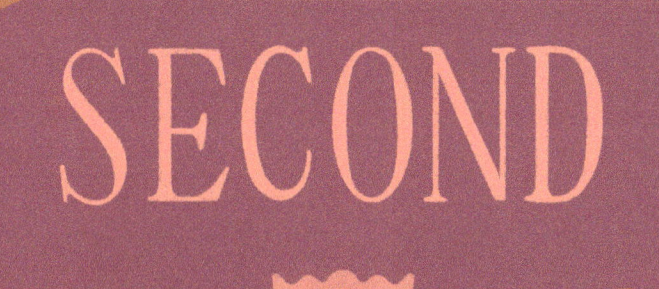

SECOND TRIMESTER

> PEOPLE ALWAYS SAY THAT PREGNANT WOMEN HAVE A *glow*. I SAY IT'S BECAUSE *you're sweating* TO DEATH.
>
> — JESSICA SIMPSON

SECOND-TRIMESTER ULTRASOUND PHOTO HERE

MONTH 4: FIRST-TIME MOM'S FIRSTS

First reaction of those you've announced your pregnancy to _____

_____
_____
_____

First flutter or kick _____

_____
_____
_____
_____

First time it really hit you that you're pregnant _____

_____
_____
_____

First unsolicited advice _____

_____
_____
_____
_____

WEEKS 13 TO 16

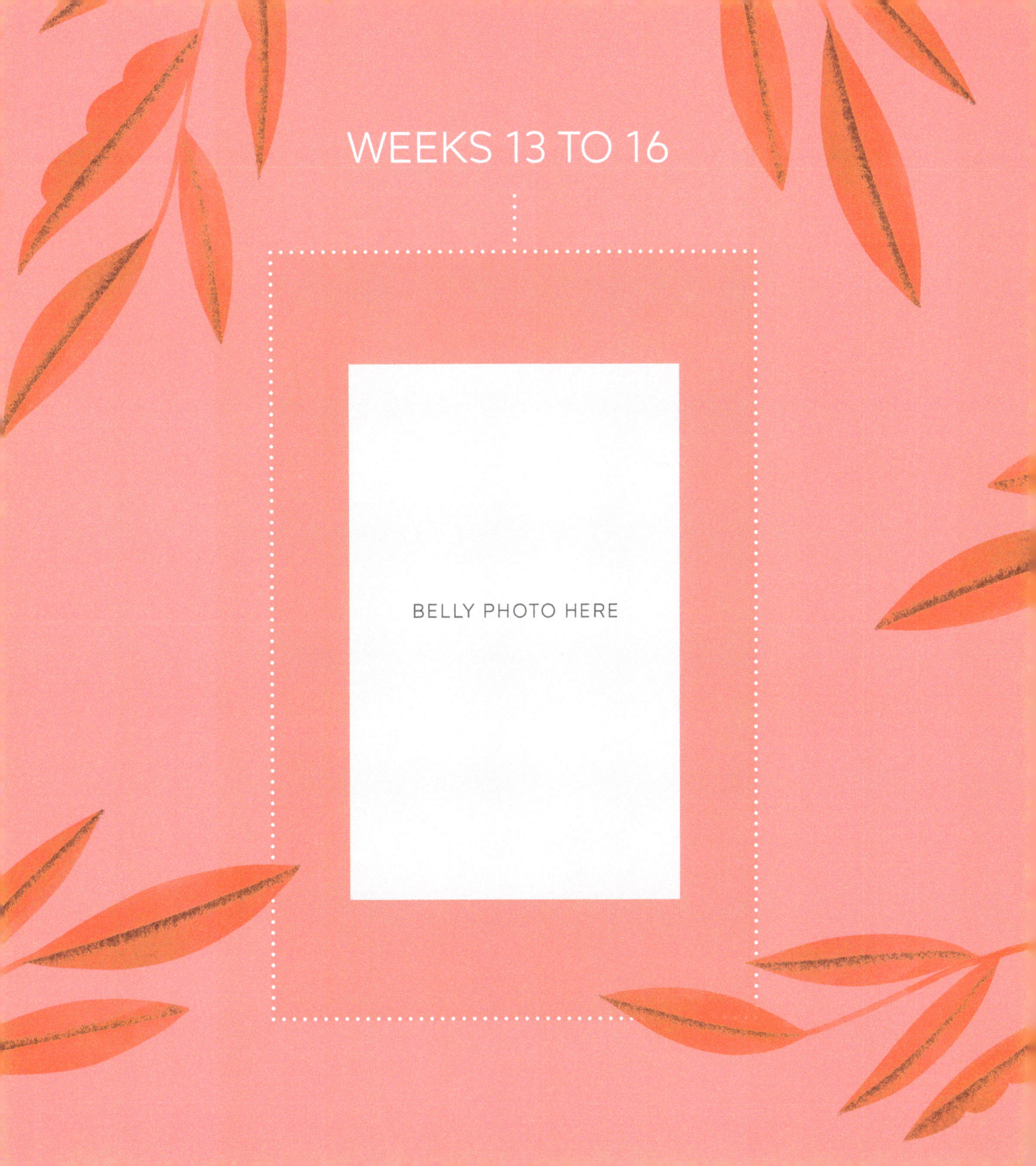

BELLY PHOTO HERE

SIZE COMPARISON

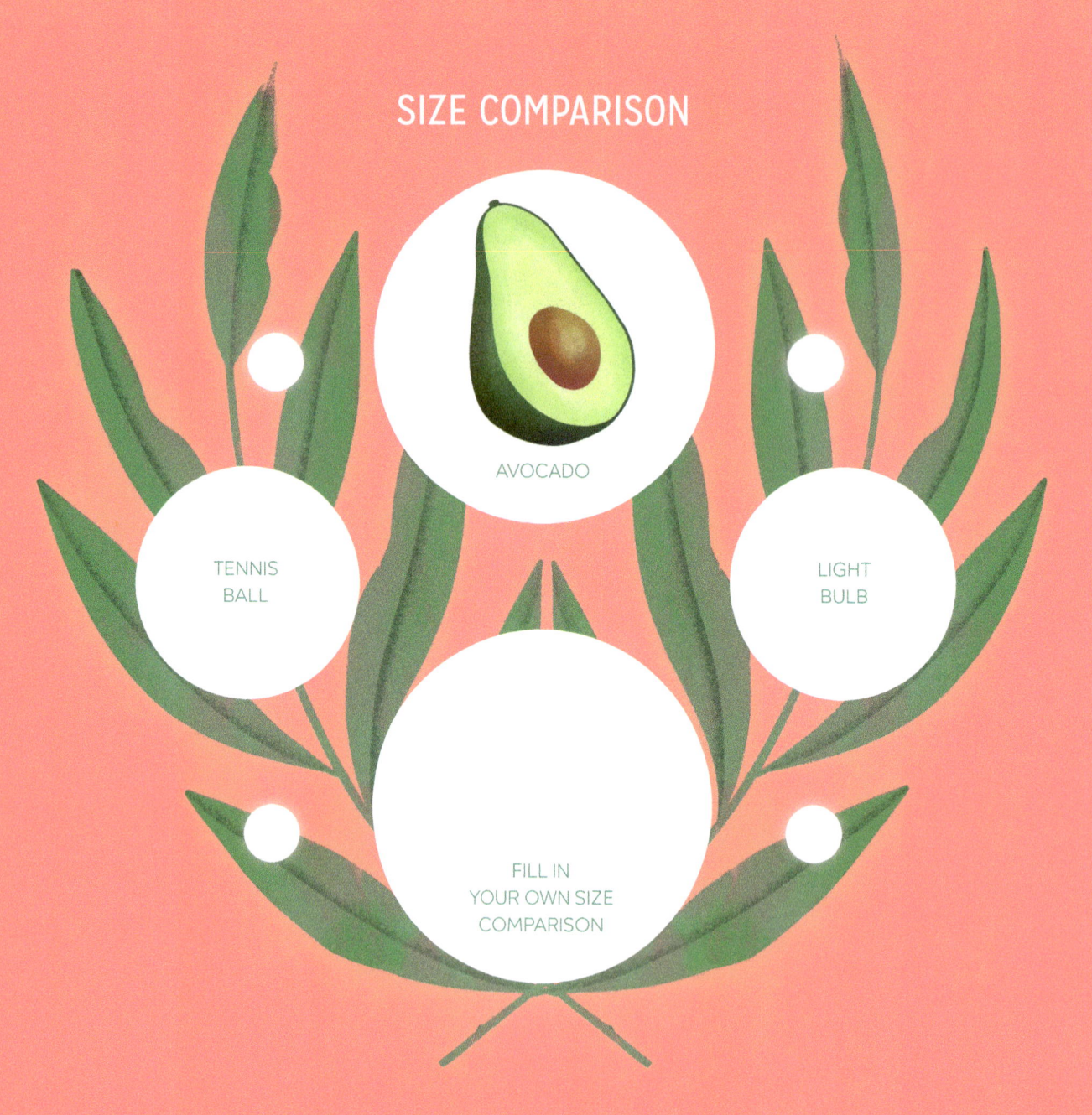

AVOCADO

TENNIS BALL

LIGHT BULB

FILL IN YOUR OWN SIZE COMPARISON

By the end of this month, your baby is about 6 inches long and weighs about 4 ounces.

PREGNANCY STATS TRACKER

Body

Have you noticed any weight gain? _____
_____

Have you experienced any itchy skin around your growing stomach or breasts? _____
_____
_____

Have you had any bloating or discomfort? _____
_____

Baby

What were your baby's stats when you went to your last prenatal appointment? _____
_____
_____
_____

How are you measuring? _____
_____

Is your due date still what it was when you first went in? If it changed, what caused your doctor/
midwife to change it? _____
_____

PRENATAL APPOINTMENTS

DATE	WEEK	WEIGHT	TESTS CONDUCTED	QUESTIONS FOR DOCTOR/MIDWIFE

MONTH 4 CHECKLIST

Home

- If you've received hand-me-down baby clothes, wash them before organizing them in drawers or a closet in the nursery (or other space you have set aside for your baby). And remember, babies don't really need much more than food, a safe place to sleep, and love. So don't sweat the small stuff or worry about having the "perfect" nursery.

- If your nesting instinct has already kicked in, take advantage of it. Keep up with everyday tasks around the house, like doing laundry, washing dishes, putting together furniture, or reorganizing closets.

- Every time you go to the grocery store, pick up one extra storable food item, such as a can of beans. This way, when you're in your first few weeks of parenthood, your pantry will be well stocked.

- Write down any house projects you need to complete before the baby comes.

- _____
- _____
- _____

Self-Care

- Schedule an appointment to get a pedicure.

- If you have an empty stomach at night, treat yourself to a midnight snack.
- Go for a walk to get some fresh air from time to time.
- _____
- _____
- _____

Baby

- Decide if you will share the name you picked out for your baby or if you will keep it a secret until the birth.
- Eat healthy foods. It takes a lot to grow a human being, and nutritious foods can only help.
- _____
- _____
- _____

Medical

- Decide now who you want in the delivery room with you so it's not a question when the birth gets closer.
- Schedule all your appointments with your doctor/midwife ahead of time so you have them on your calendar.

- If you are on a payment plan with your doctor/midwife, make sure to make timely payments and have a plan to pay the full amount as soon as you are able.
- _____
- _____
- _____

Important Events

- Now that you're in your second trimester, make a plan to announce your pregnancy to people you haven't told yet.
- If a gender-reveal event is in your plans, schedule when you want to do it.
- If you have a significant other, plan a "babymoon"—a time for you to get away before the baby is born.
- _____
- _____
- _____

DAILY REMINDERS

○	○	○
Drink 10 cups of water over the course of the day.	Take your prenatal vitamin.	Eat at least three meals and three snacks.

Activity #1

Write a list of people in your life who inspire and uplift you. Shoot them a text to thank them for their light and give them a genuine compliment. Sometimes during pregnancy we forget to be a good friend to others, so take the time to thank those who are there for you. If there isn't anyone specific, reach out to someone you would like to be closer to.

_____
_____
_____
_____
_____
_____
_____
_____
_____
_____

Activity #2

Make a gratitude list of everything you are thankful for today.

_____
_____
_____
_____
_____
_____
_____
_____
_____
_____
_____
_____
_____

Activity #3

Write down five words you think will describe you as a parent.

....

....

....

....

....

Activity #4

Write "I got this" several times down the page, and then repeat it out loud. You were made for this pregnancy, and your body is made to give birth.

Gratitude

What person in your life have you felt extra grateful for lately and why?

_____
_____
_____
_____
_____

Challenge

What have you been struggling with most this month—physically or emotionally?

_____
_____
_____
_____
_____

Reflection

What has happened so far this month to make you feel extra special?

_____
_____
_____
_____
_____

Observation

What has been filling your mind during this part of your pregnancy? Any worries? Expectations? Fears? Excitement?

_____
_____
_____
_____
_____

FREESTYLE JOURNAL

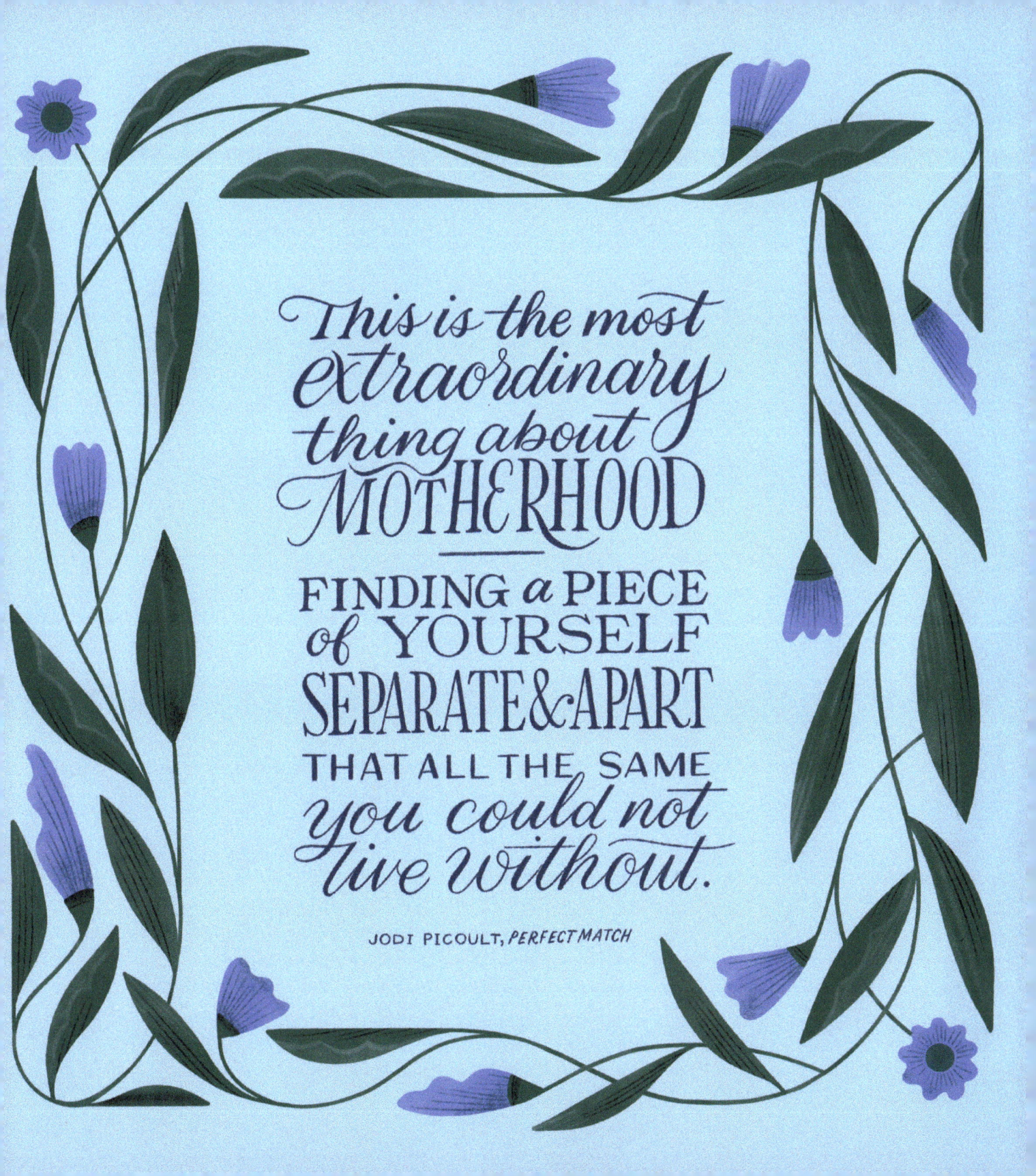

This is the most extraordinary thing about MOTHERHOOD —

FINDING a PIECE of YOURSELF SEPARATE & APART THAT ALL THE SAME *you could not live without.*

JODI PICOULT, *PERFECT MATCH*

MONTH 5: FIRST-TIME MOM'S FIRSTS

First day you felt a little more energy _____

First time you accidentally peed a little when you sneezed _____

First time someone asked when you were due _____

First person you noticed (on social media or in your circle of friends) who is also pregnant _____

First good night's sleep _____

WEEKS 17 TO 20

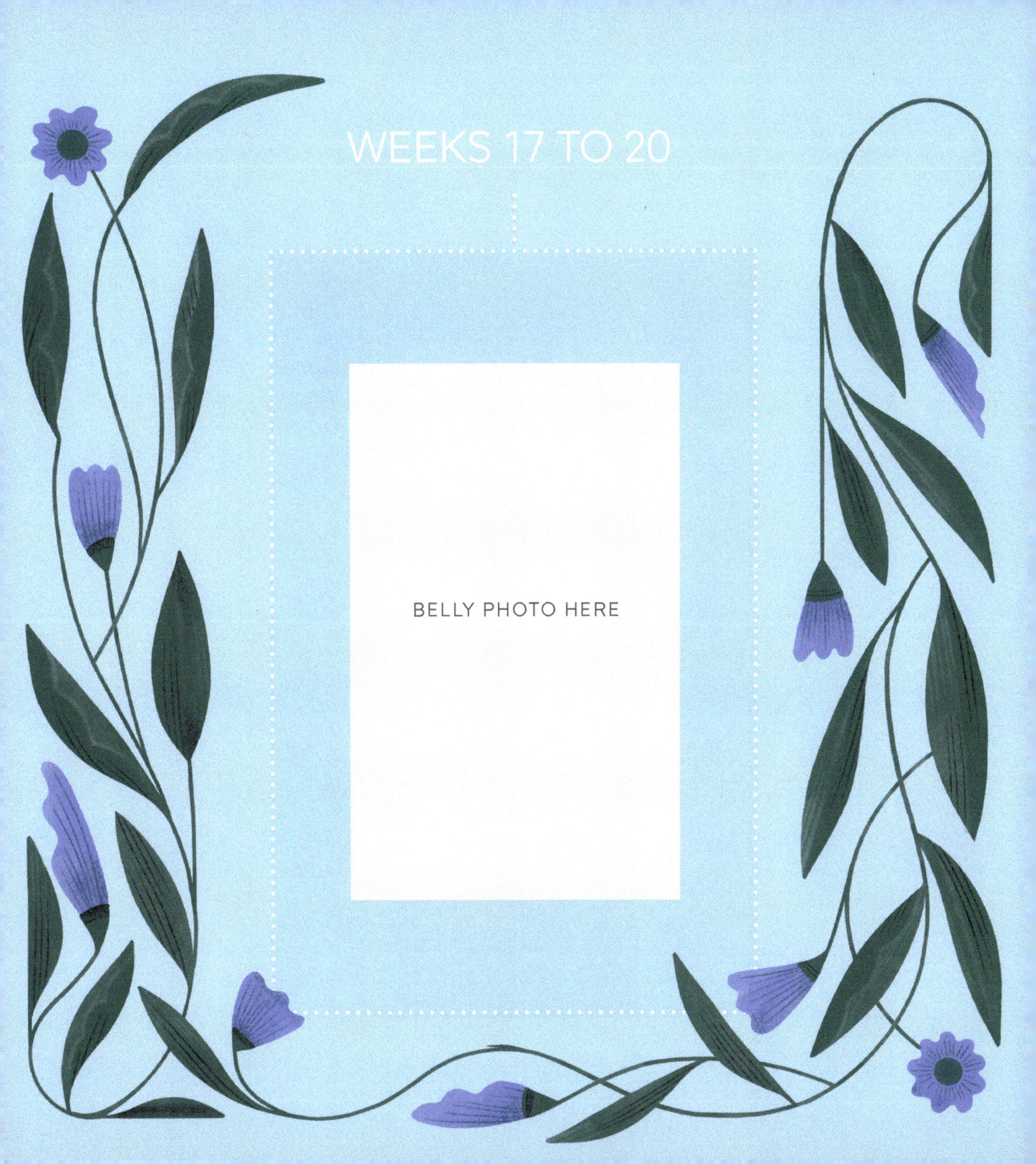

BELLY PHOTO HERE

SIZE COMPARISON

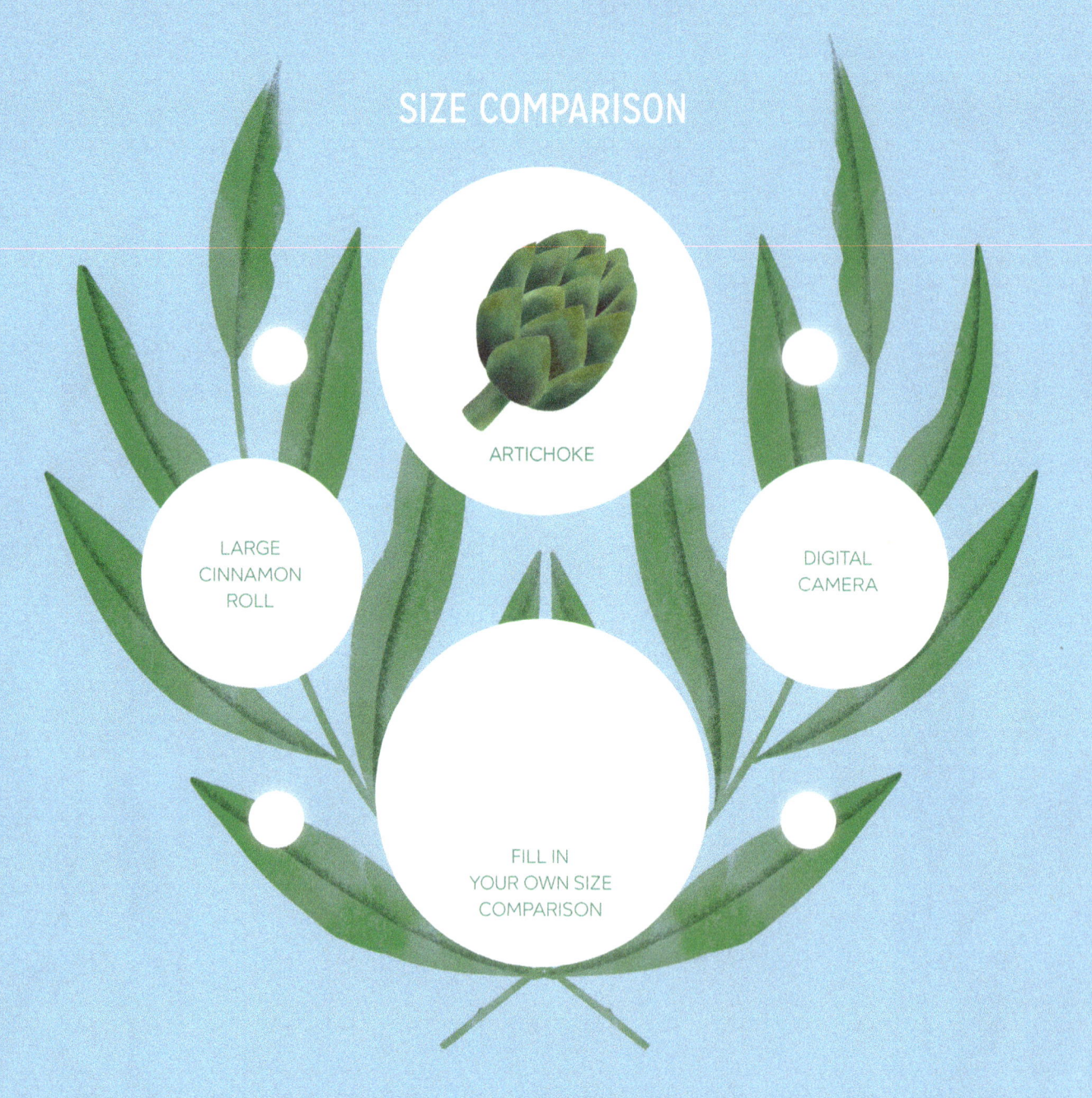

ARTICHOKE

LARGE CINNAMON ROLL

DIGITAL CAMERA

FILL IN YOUR OWN SIZE COMPARISON

By the end of this month, your baby is about 10 inches long and weighs about 1 pound.

PREGNANCY STATS TRACKER

Body

Your blood pressure, blood volume, and heart rate are changing constantly; have you noticed a drop in blood pressure or an increased heart rate? _____

_____

How is your appetite? _____

_____

How is your energy? _____

_____

Any dizzy spells? _____

_____

Baby

Were there any surprises (such as twins) at your 20-week ultrasound? _____

_____

_____

At this point, your baby has eyebrows, eyelashes, hair, and tiny teeth. How is your baby measuring?
_____
_____

What is your official due date? _____
_____

Did you find out your baby's gender? _____
_____

PRENATAL APPOINTMENTS

DATE	WEEK	WEIGHT	TESTS CONDUCTED	QUESTIONS FOR DOCTOR/MIDWIFE

MONTH 5 CHECKLIST

Home

- ○ Set up the crib, if you have one.
- ○ Organize any new baby-related items you've gotten in the past month.
- ○ If the baby will be sleeping in your bedroom at first, decide how you will rearrange the furniture to make room for the crib or bassinet.
- ○ Ask for help moving heavy items so you don't have to lift anything yourself.
- ○ _____
- ○ _____
- ○ _____

Self-Care

- Go out with your girlfriends. Pretty soon movies, plays, and dinners out will be harder to attend, so soak up all that girl time!
- Sleep as often as you can. Remember, babies need to eat every two to three hours at first, so in a few months sleep will feel like gold!
- If your nausea has gone away, try to eat smaller but more frequent meals. You'll find your body will feel better than it does when you indulge in larger meals.
- _____
- _____
- _____

Baby

- Buy a decorative memento box that you can fill with items and information about your baby to share with them in later years.
- If you've been dreaming about a certain large-ticket item, such as a stroller, hold off on buying it until after a baby shower. You'll want to avoid getting duplicate items—unless you're having twins.
- _____
- _____
- _____

Medical

- Gather all your medical records and documents and put them in a folder for easy access. Include ultrasound pictures and medical history documents.
- _____
- _____
- _____

Important Events

- Confirm the date of your baby shower and create your baby gift registry.
- _____
- _____
- _____

DAILY REMINDERS

- Drink 10 cups of water over the course of the day.
- Take your prenatal vitamin.
- Eat at least three meals and three snacks.

Activity #1

Take a walk outside, breathe some fresh air,

or sit on your porch for five minutes.

Think about what brings you joy, and then write it down.

_____

_____

_____

_____

_____

_____

_____

_____

_____

_____

_____

_____

Activity #2

Research mom support groups and write down a few you would like to join. Also check out the Mamahood Blog community on Facebook or Instagram to get started.

Activity #3

Make a list of your personality traits.

Circle all the traits you think your baby will have.

Activity #4

Create a mood/color board with color swatches, fabric samples, and other inspiration for decorating your nursery.

Gratitude

Who has been your biggest supporter? Brainstorm ways to express your gratitude to them.

_____
_____
_____
_____
_____
_____

Challenge

Has one or more of your relationships changed in big or subtle ways since you announced that you are pregnant? If so, how?

_____
_____
_____
_____
_____

Reflection

What's been your favorite place to hang out since learning you were pregnant? Why do you like to be there?

_____
_____
_____
_____
_____

Observation

What have the people around you said about your pregnancy? How do you think they feel?

_____
_____
_____
_____
_____

FREESTYLE JOURNAL

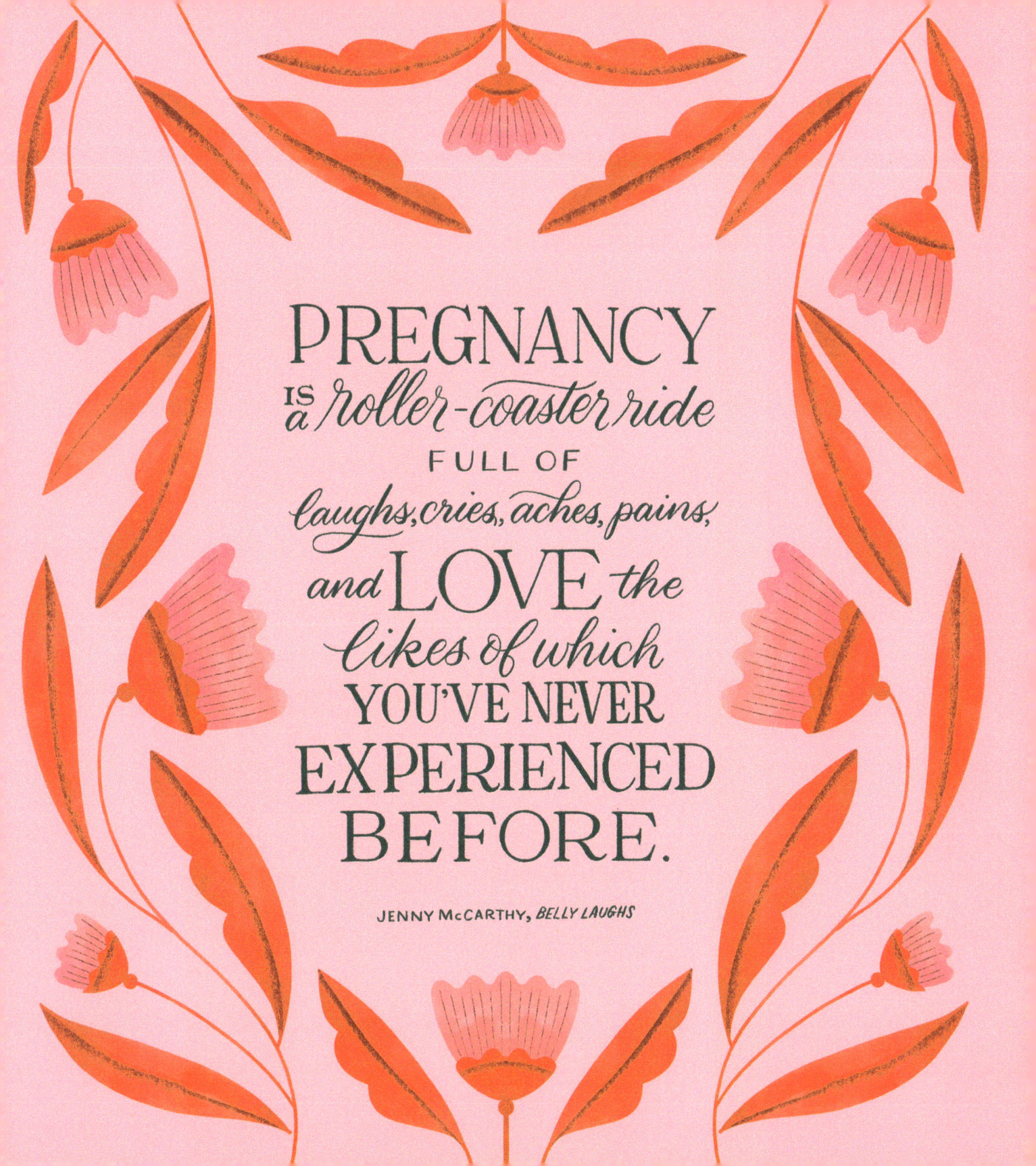

PREGNANCY IS a roller-coaster ride FULL OF laughs, cries, aches, pains, and LOVE the likes of which YOU'VE NEVER EXPERIENCED BEFORE.

JENNY McCARTHY, *BELLY LAUGHS*

MONTH 6: FIRST-TIME MOM'S FIRSTS

First time the baby kicked you in the ribs _____

First awkward moment with your doctor/midwife _____

First impression of your new belly button _____

First connection or bonding you felt with your baby, if any _____

First time someone offered to lift something for you or gave up their seat for you _____

WEEKS 21 TO 24

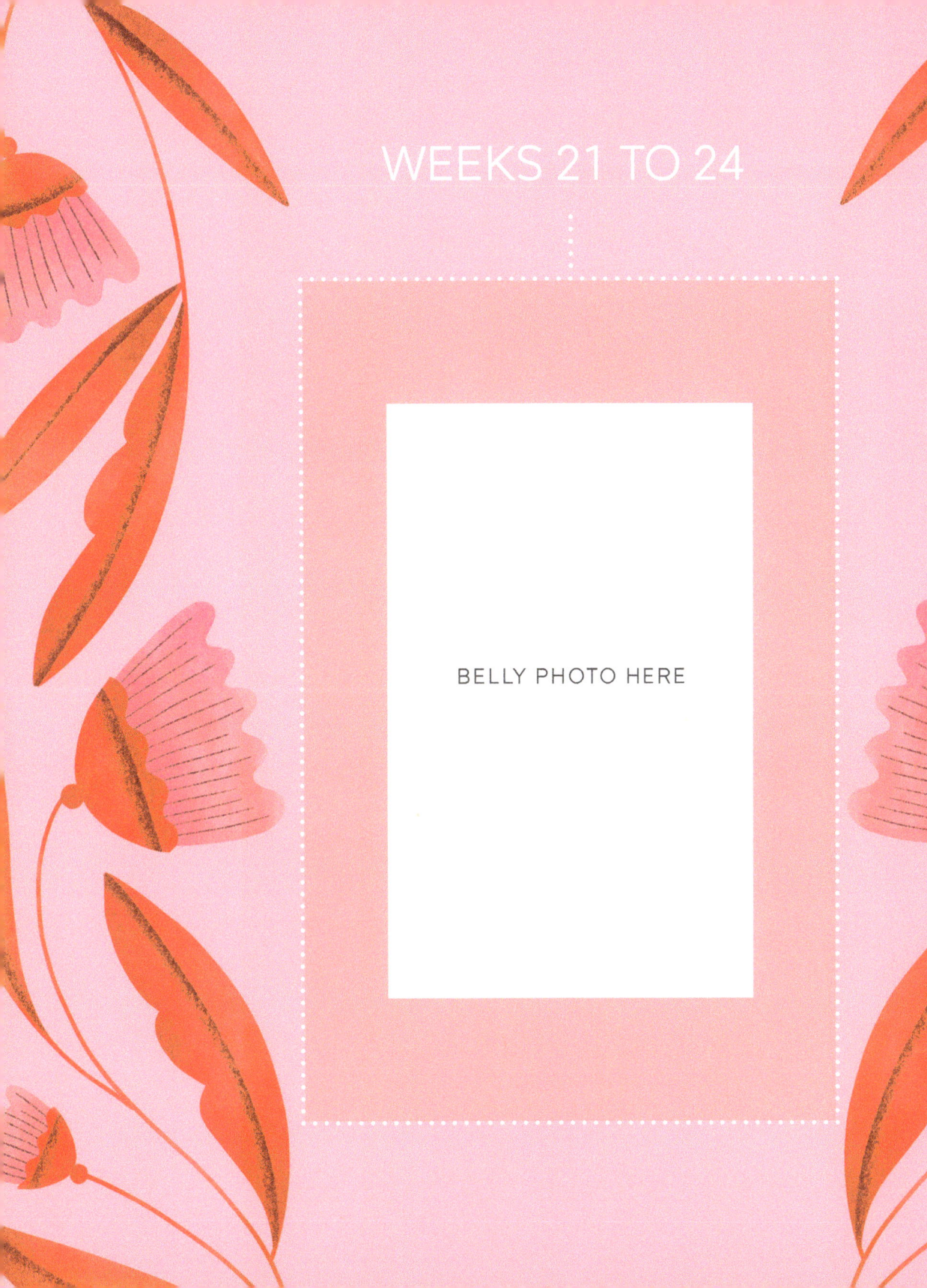

BELLY PHOTO HERE

SIZE COMPARISON

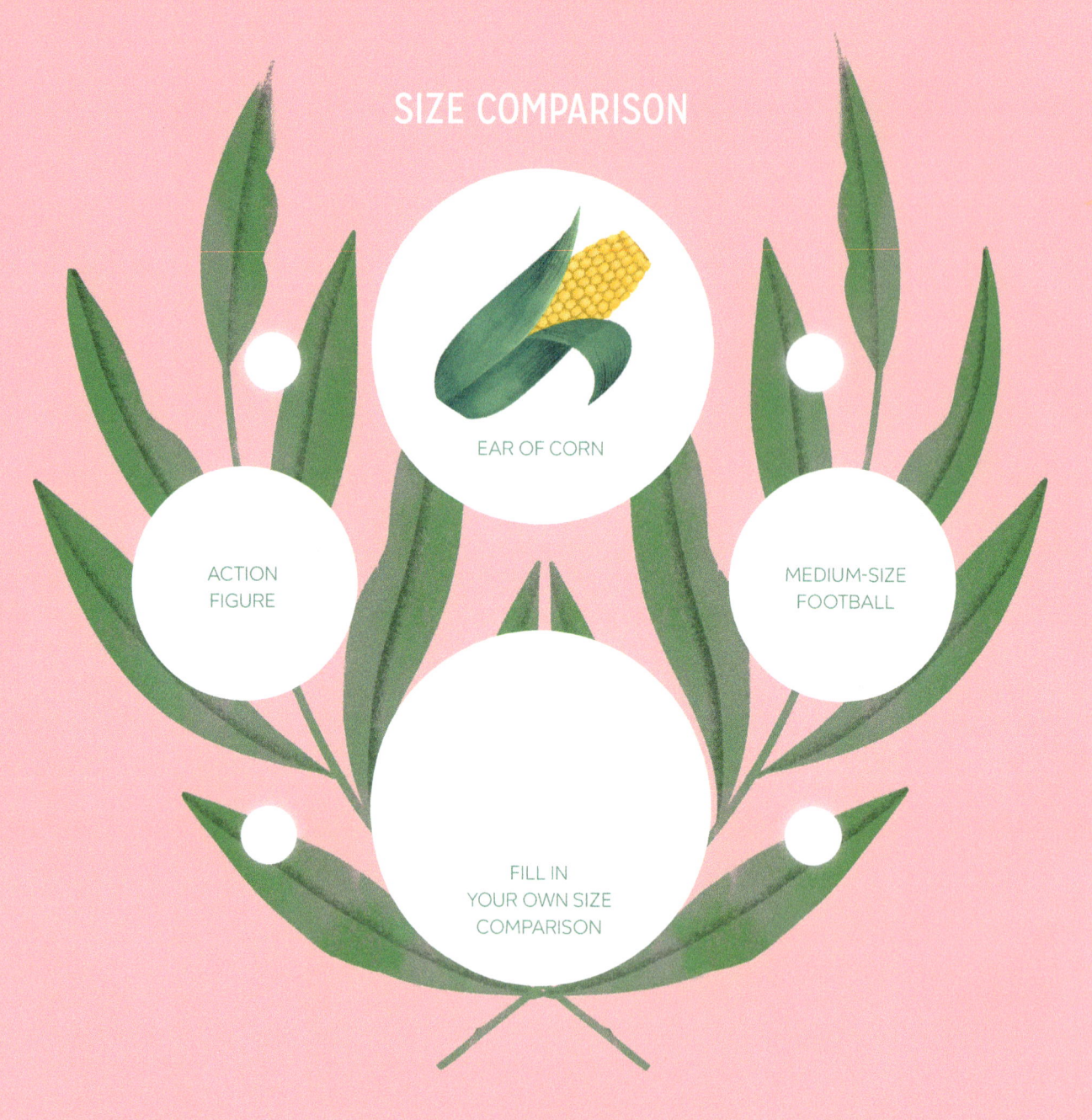

EAR OF CORN

ACTION FIGURE

MEDIUM-SIZE FOOTBALL

FILL IN YOUR OWN SIZE COMPARISON

By the end of this month, your baby is about 12 inches long and weighs about 2 pounds.

PREGNANCY STATS TRACKER

Body

Your body might start to retain water. Have you noticed any swelling? _____

Do you feel a little bit squished yet? _____

Your baby has taste buds now and might react to different foods you eat. Have you noticed any changes when you eat spicy foods? _____

Have you had any constipation recently, or are things smooth sailing? _____

Have you noticed the appearance of any stretch marks? _____

Baby

Your baby's lungs are developing. Were you able to spot them on the ultrasound at your last

prenatal appointment? _____
_____

How are your baby's growth patterns? _____
_____

Have there been any health scares or problems so far? _____
_____

PRENATAL APPOINTMENTS

DATE	WEEK	WEIGHT	TESTS CONDUCTED	QUESTIONS FOR DOCTOR/MIDWIFE

MONTH 6 CHECKLIST

Home

- Finish any major projects in your home.
- Start thinking about what kind of rules/values you want in your home.
- Create a safe environment for you and your baby. Make sure to buy baby-proofing gear for electrical outlets, cabinet doors, cords, stairs, and other potential hazards, and install the gear before the baby arrives.
- Figure out which chair in your home you will use to rock your baby.
- _____
- _____
- _____

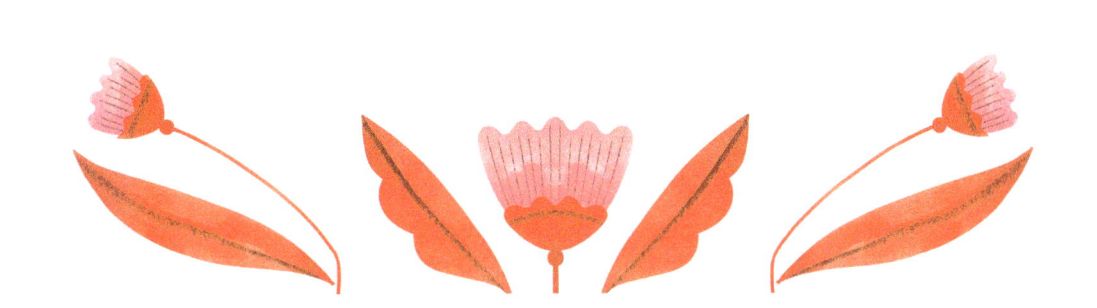

Self-Care

- Spend time doing your favorite thing. You'll still be able to enjoy your favorite thing once the baby arrives; it will just be a little trickier.
- Spending too much time on your feet might start to get uncomfortable. Put your feet up during the day if your schedule allows it.
- Make sure to find your tribe or a support person you can talk to about the big and little things.
- You're eating for two (or maybe more), so treat yourself to a tasty dessert every once in a while.
- Find yourself a good pair of maternity jeans. They are so worth it!
- _____
- _____
- _____

Baby

- Decide if you are going to breastfeed or formula feed. If you have concerns, talk to your doctor/midwife about this decision. Also remember that your baby might not be able to eat exactly how you dream they will, so allow yourself to be flexible and have a plan B. No mama should ever feel guilty about how she feeds her baby. Fed is best.
- Do your research on different birth preferences. Is there anything specific you want for the baby at delivery? Delayed cord clamping? Waiting 24 hours for a bath?
- Get your baby shower on the calendar.
- Look at what baby items you already have and finalize your baby-gift registry.
- _____
- _____
- _____

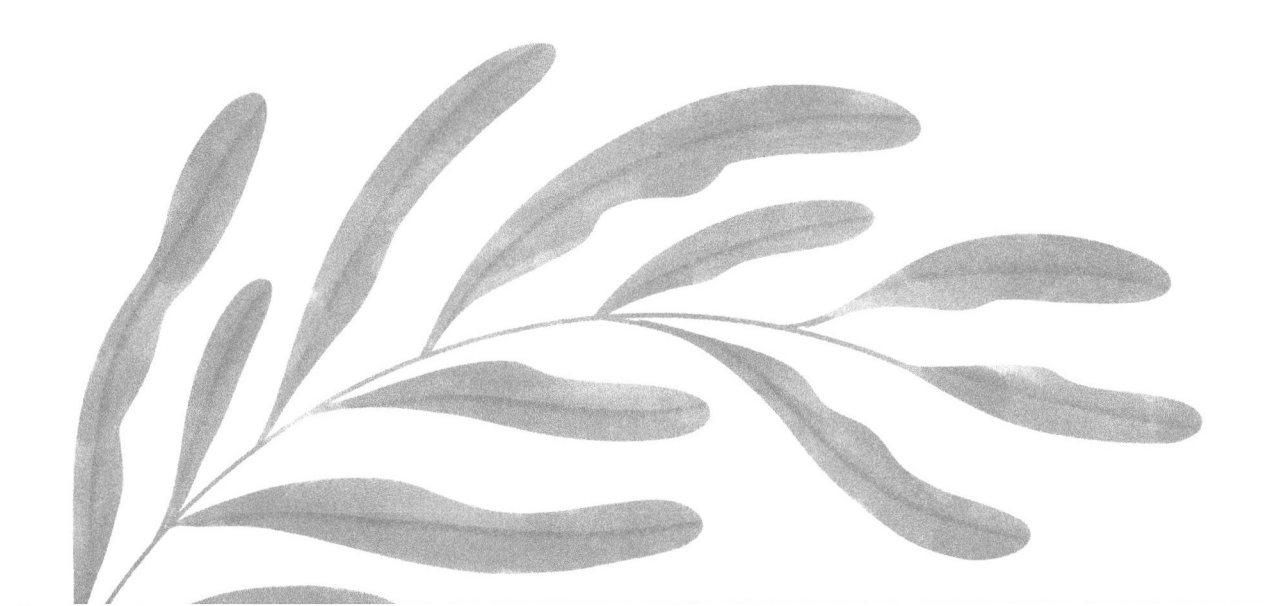

Medical

- Start writing out your birth plan.
- Take a tour of the hospital where you will be delivering.
- Ask your doctor/midwife any questions you have about delivery or the anticipated timeline.
- Review again who you would like to be in the delivery room, and talk to them about your expectations about delivery.
- _____
- _____
- _____

Important Events

- Decide if you want maternity or birth pictures.
- If you are going to take that babymoon, right now is a great time. Just make sure to clear it with your doctor/midwife, and go before it's too late.
- Check to see if there are any pop-up shops or sales going on this month to help you stock up on baby items. If you are having a shower, you will get a lot of needed items, but it's still fun to shop for your tiny bundle yourself, too.
- _____
- _____
- _____

DAILY REMINDERS

- Drink 10 cups of water over the course of the day.
- Take your prenatal vitamin.
- Eat at least three meals and three snacks.

Activity #1

Make a bucket list of all the things
you want to do before the baby comes.

Activity #2

On a scale of 1 to 10, with 10 being the most stressed, how are you feeling right now about becoming a mom? Circle the number below. Write about the level of stress you are feeling.

_____
_____
_____
_____
_____
_____
_____
_____
_____

1 2 3 4 5 6 7 8 9 10

Activity #3

Write down five things you have loved about being pregnant this month. Then write down five things you have disliked.

WHAT I LOVED	WHAT I DISLIKED

Activity #4

If you have a name picked out,
write down what the name means to you.

_____
_____
_____
_____
_____
_____
_____
_____
_____

....

Baby's Name

Gratitude

How did you feel when you found out the gender of your baby, if you chose to find out?

_____
_____
_____
_____

Challenge

Have you been having difficulty sleeping at night? Describe a usual night.

_____
_____
_____
_____
_____

Reflection

Does your baby seem to have a personality yet? If so, what's it like?

_____
_____
_____
_____
_____

Observation

What was it like the first time you felt your baby kick? Does your baby kick a lot during the day or night? What other movements have you been feeling? Any hiccups?

_____
_____
_____
_____
_____

FREESTYLE JOURNAL

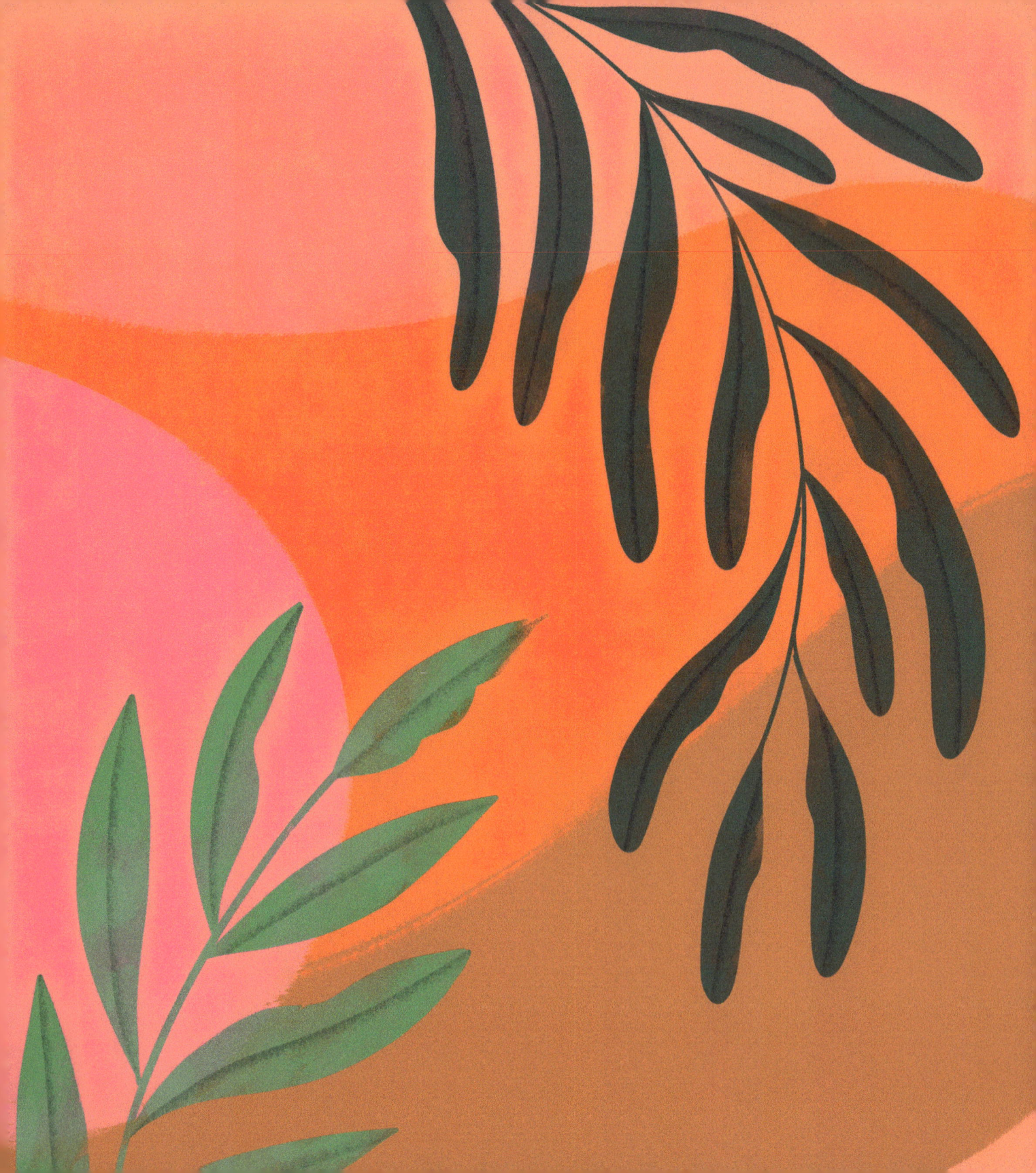

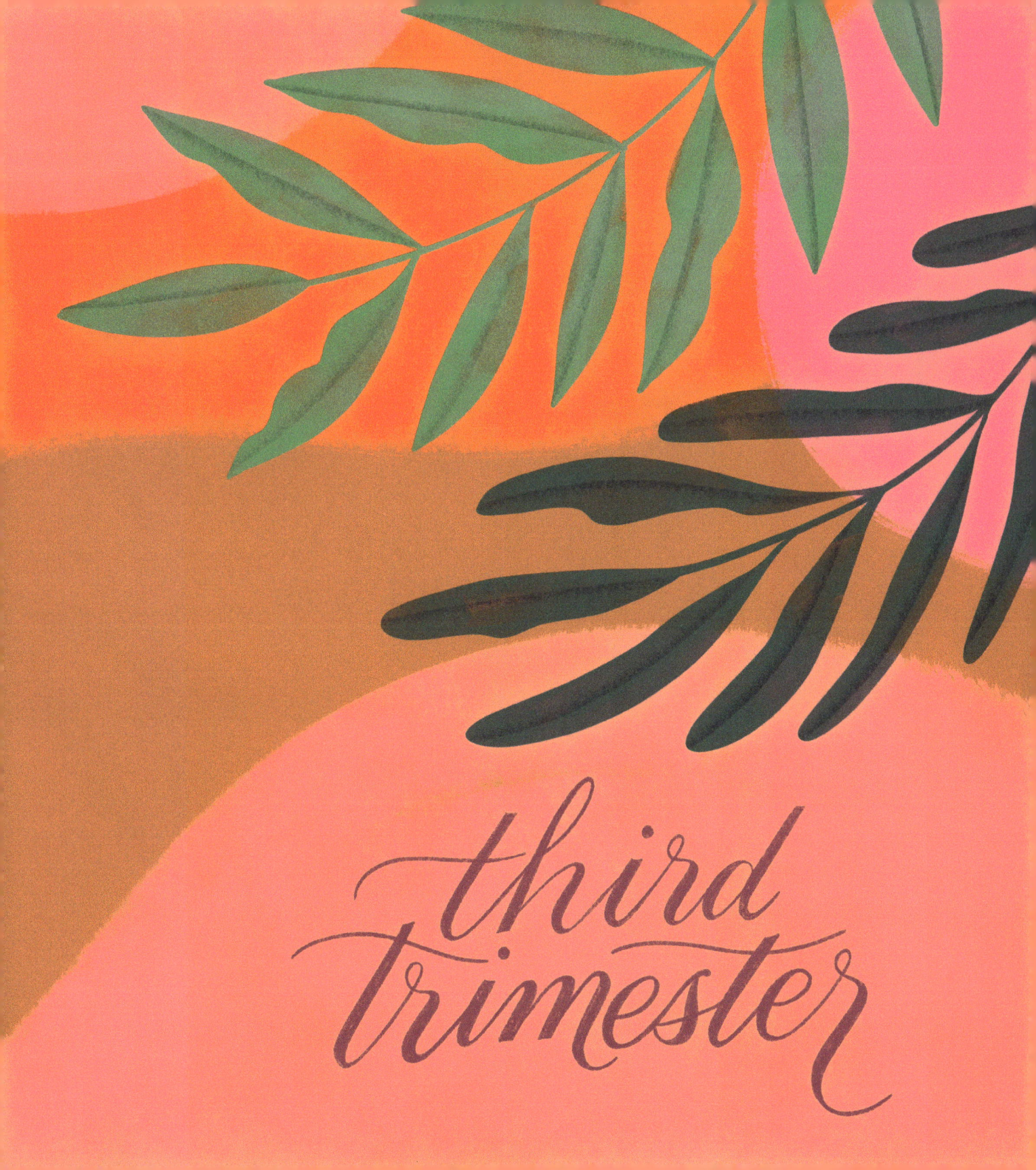

third trimester

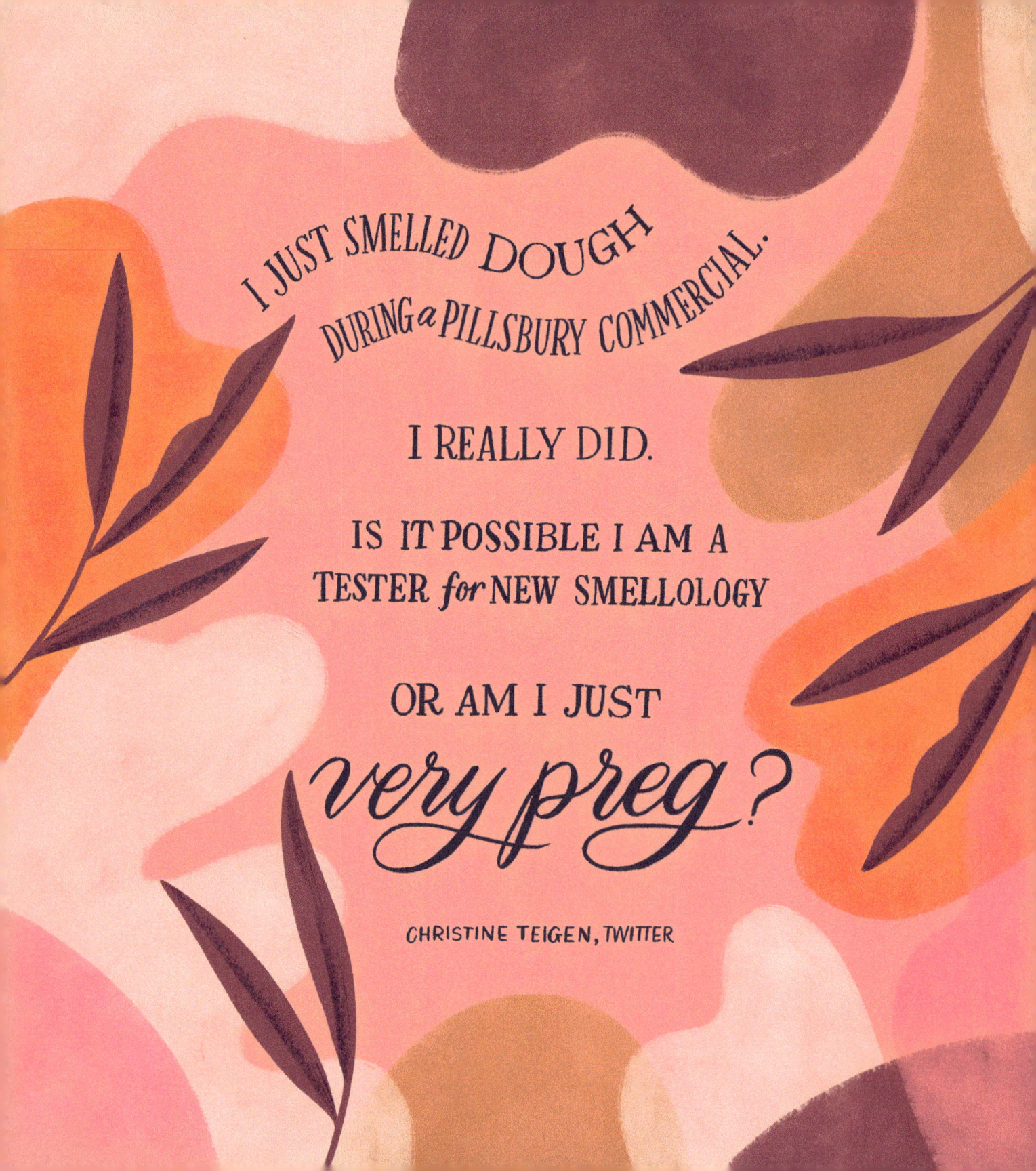

I JUST SMELLED DOUGH DURING a PILLSBURY COMMERCIAL.

I REALLY DID.

IS IT POSSIBLE I AM A TESTER *for* NEW SMELLOLOGY

OR AM I JUST *very preg*?

CHRISTINE TEIGEN, TWITTER

THIRD-TRIMESTER ULTRASOUND

PHOTO HERE

MONTH 7: FIRST-TIME MOM'S FIRSTS

First time you felt comfortable in your pregnant body _____

_____

_____

_____

First question you asked other moms you know _____

_____

_____

_____

First thing you think you will miss about being pregnant _____

_____

_____

_____

First pregnancy brain moment _____

_____

_____

First time a stranger touched your belly _____

_____

_____

WEEKS 25 TO 28

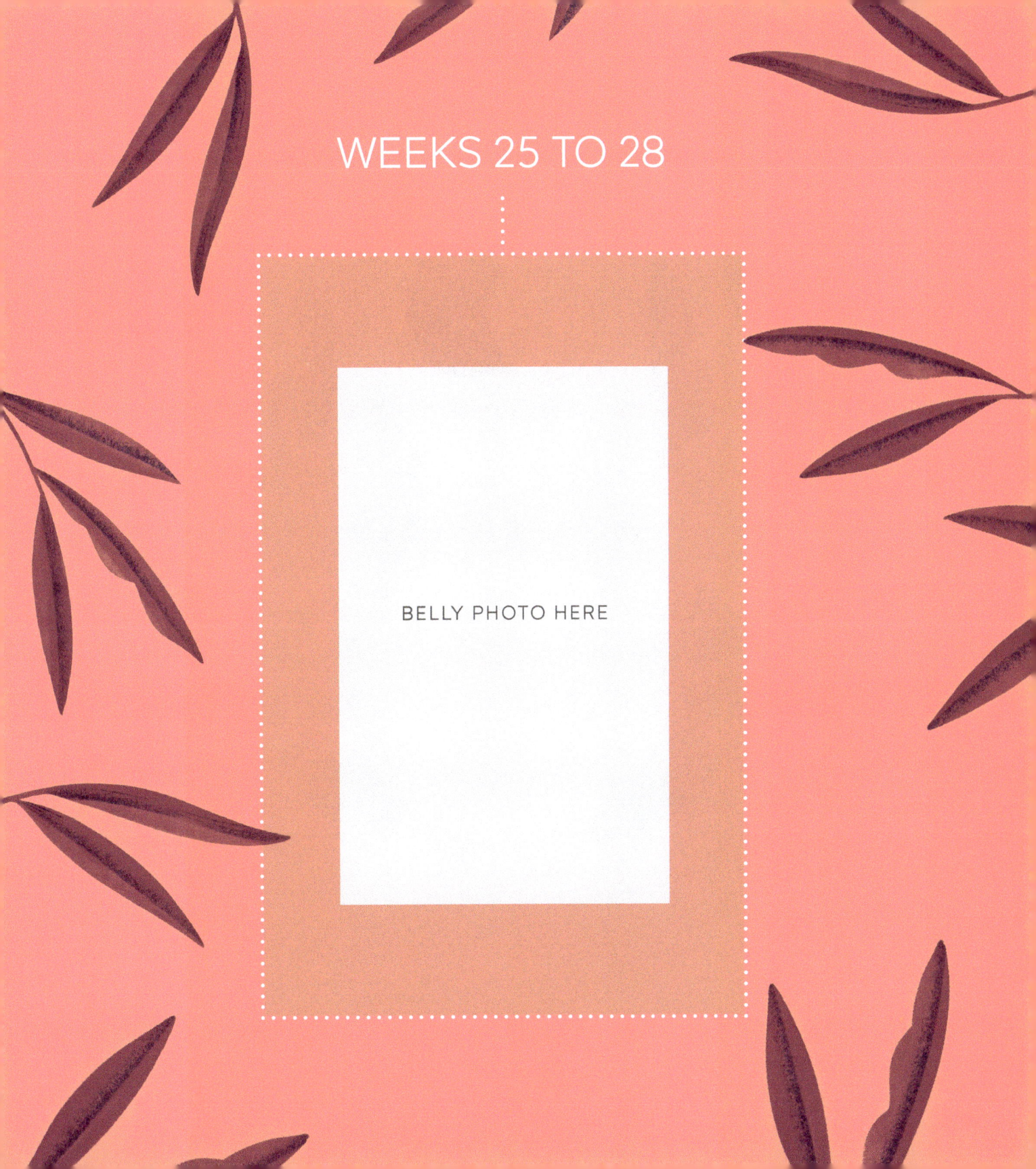

BELLY PHOTO HERE

SIZE COMPARISON

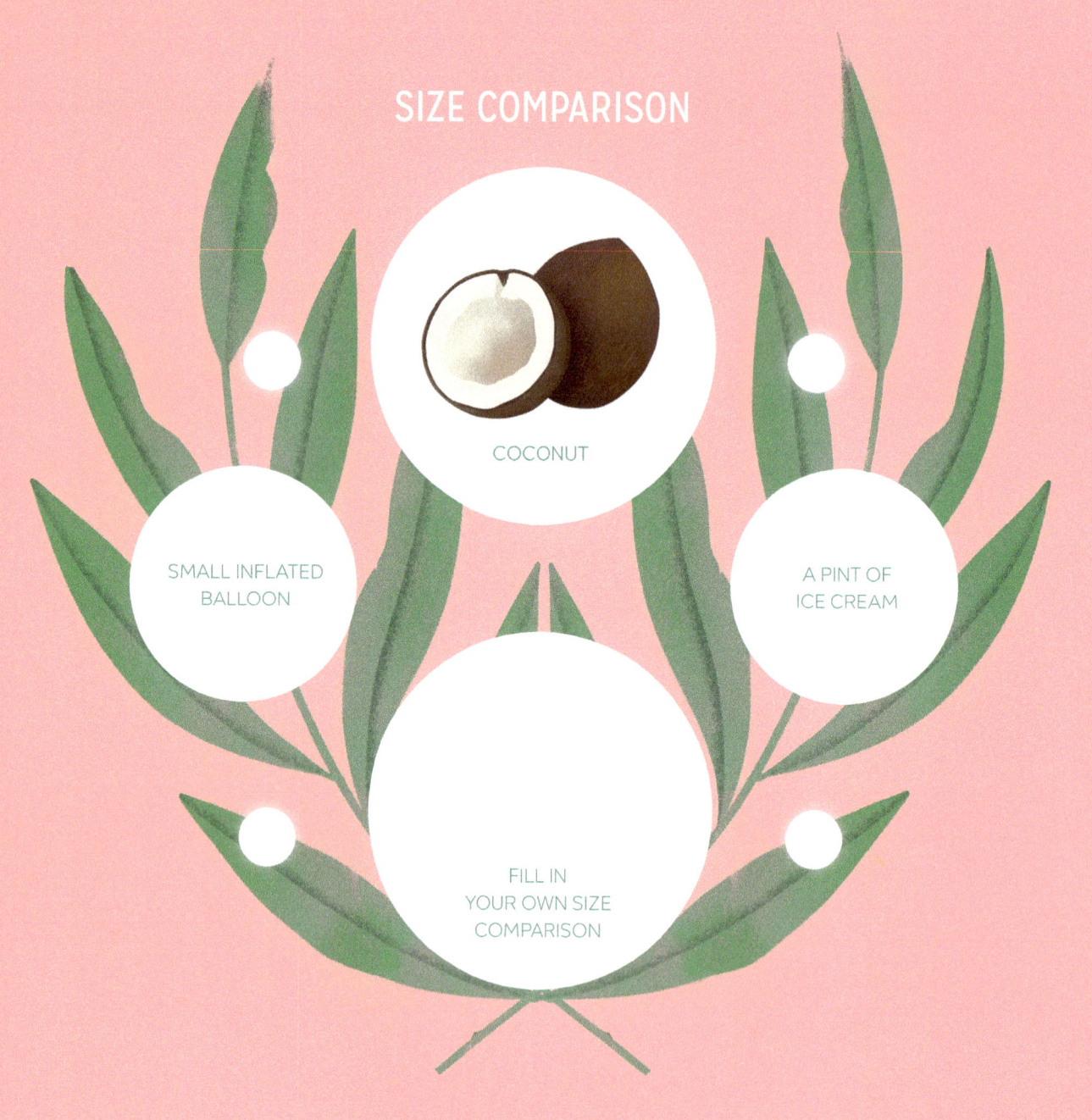

COCONUT

SMALL INFLATED BALLOON

A PINT OF ICE CREAM

FILL IN YOUR OWN SIZE COMPARISON

By the end of this month, your baby is about 14 inches long and weighs 2 to 4 pounds.

PREGNANCY STATS TRACKER

Body

Are you feeling your baby kicking and wiggling more frequently? You are probably feeling all sorts of movement by now and are getting used to having a little buddy with you 24/7. _____
_____

Have you had any back pain? _____
_____

Do you feel like you can't eat a lot because your stomach is getting squished? _____
_____

Have you had any shortness of breath? _____
_____

Have you noticed any changes with your breasts as your body is getting ready to lactate? Some women will observe colostrum early on. _____
_____

Baby

Has your doctor or midwife been able to tell you the position of your baby yet? _____
_____

Does your baby seem active at certain times of the day or night? _____
_____

Your baby's hands should be fully developed. Have you been able to have another ultrasound lately? What details stood out to you most from that ultrasound? _____
_____

PRENATAL APPOINTMENTS

DATE	WEEK	WEIGHT	TESTS CONDUCTED	QUESTIONS FOR DOCTOR/MIDWIFE

MONTH 7 CHECKLIST

Home

- Map out exactly where you want to place everything in the nursery.
- Find pictures to hang on the nursery walls.
- If you have items that need to be assembled, such as a stroller, put them together now.
- Get some bins that fit in a closet or dresser so you can organize clothes and accessories.
- _____
- _____
- _____

Self-Care

- You might start to notice times when your baby is less active or sleeping. Try to sleep during those times, if your schedule allows.
- If you are having back problems, consider seeing a chiropractor or prenatal massage therapist.
- Tell your significant other or any close friends or family when you are tired, uncomfortable, or hurting.
- _____

- _____
- _____

Baby

- Count kicks every day, and if anything feels off with regard to your baby's activity, speak to your doctor/midwife.
- Understand how to recognize a Braxton Hicks contraction.
- Make sure to get your glucose tolerance test done by the time you are 28 weeks pregnant. This test screens for gestational diabetes.
- Get a "take home" outfit for your baby to wear on the way home from the hospital.
- _____
- _____
- _____

Medical

- Start talking to your doctor/midwife about what you expect at delivery and review your preferences.
- Review your birth plan and make adjustments as needed.

- Attend a childbirth education class with your significant other or close friend or family member to help you know what to expect, and gain some confidence, knowledge, and excitement about giving birth.

- _____
- _____
- _____

Important Events

- If you've decided to have maternity pictures taken, schedule the photo shoot now. Be sure to have it before you hit the 35-week mark, after which you may feel too big or too swollen.

- Book a birth photographer, birth videographer, and/or newborn photographer, if you'd like to have your delivery documented in one of these ways.

- _____
- _____
- _____

DAILY REMINDERS

- Drink 10 cups of water over the course of the day.
- Take your prenatal vitamin.
- Eat at least three meals and three snacks.

Activity #1

Search "birth affirmations" online, and fill up the page with your favorites. Then read them out loud.

_____
_____
_____
_____
_____
_____
_____
_____
_____
_____
_____
_____

Activity #2

Write one "strength" word in the middle of this page.
It could be "brave," "empower," "strong," or some other word
that speaks to you. Then write what that word means to you.
Each night, when you go to sleep, think about that word and everything
it evokes until you believe that you are embodying that word 100 percent.

....

Strength Word

Activity #3

If you have a significant other, list your expectations and your significant other's in the respective circles in the diagram below. Put your shared expectations in the middle of the diagram, where the circles overlap.

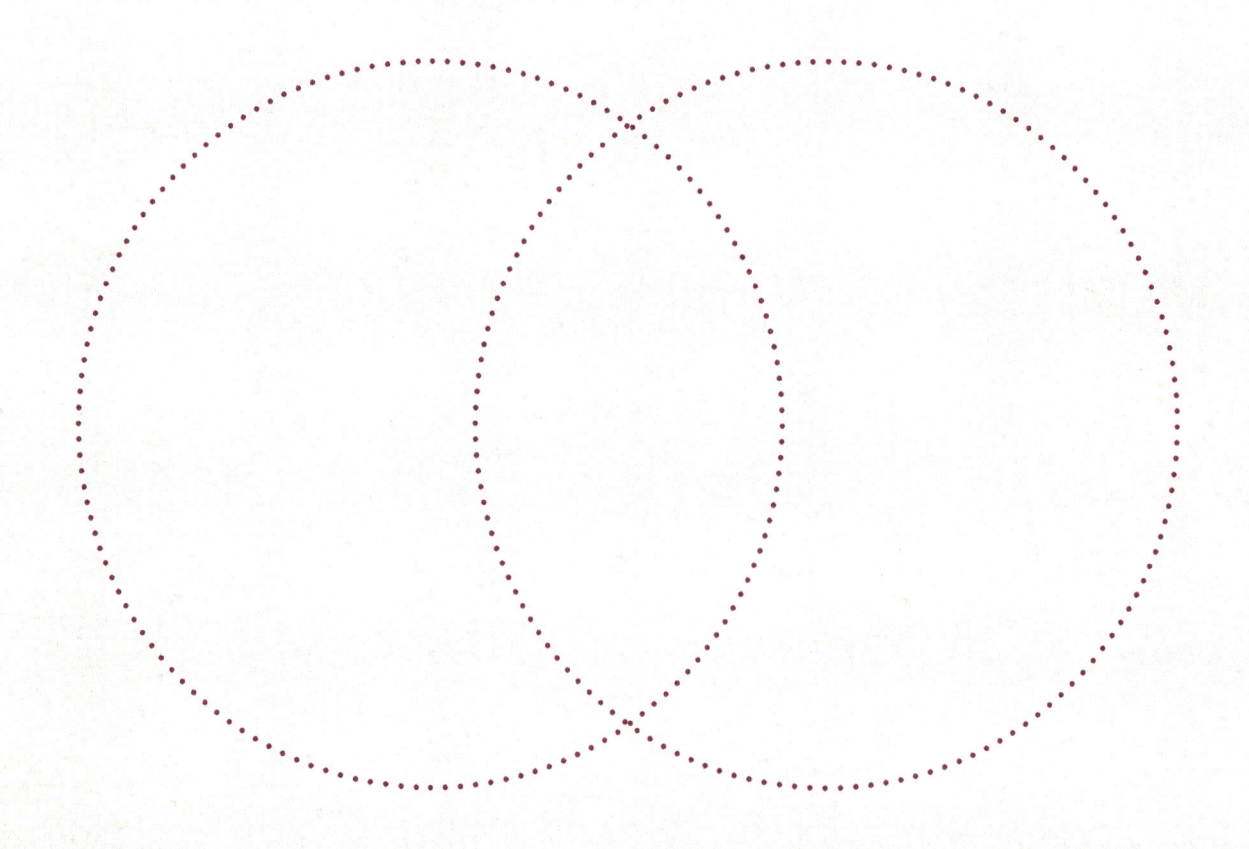

Activity #4

In the first column, list any worries or fears you have about giving birth.
In the second column, list ways to overcome those worries or fears,
as well as people who can help you overcome them.

MY WORRIES AND FEARS	WAYS TO OVERCOME THEM OR PEOPLE WHO CAN HELP

Gratitude

After you left your last appointment with your doctor/midwife, what, if anything, were you thankful for?

_____
_____
_____
_____

Challenge

What's been the hardest pregnancy symptom for you this month?

_____
_____
_____
_____

Reflection

What do you look forward to most about becoming a mom?

_____
_____
_____
_____
_____

Observation

Will you miss being pregnant? Why or why not?

_____
_____
_____
_____
_____

FREESTYLE JOURNAL

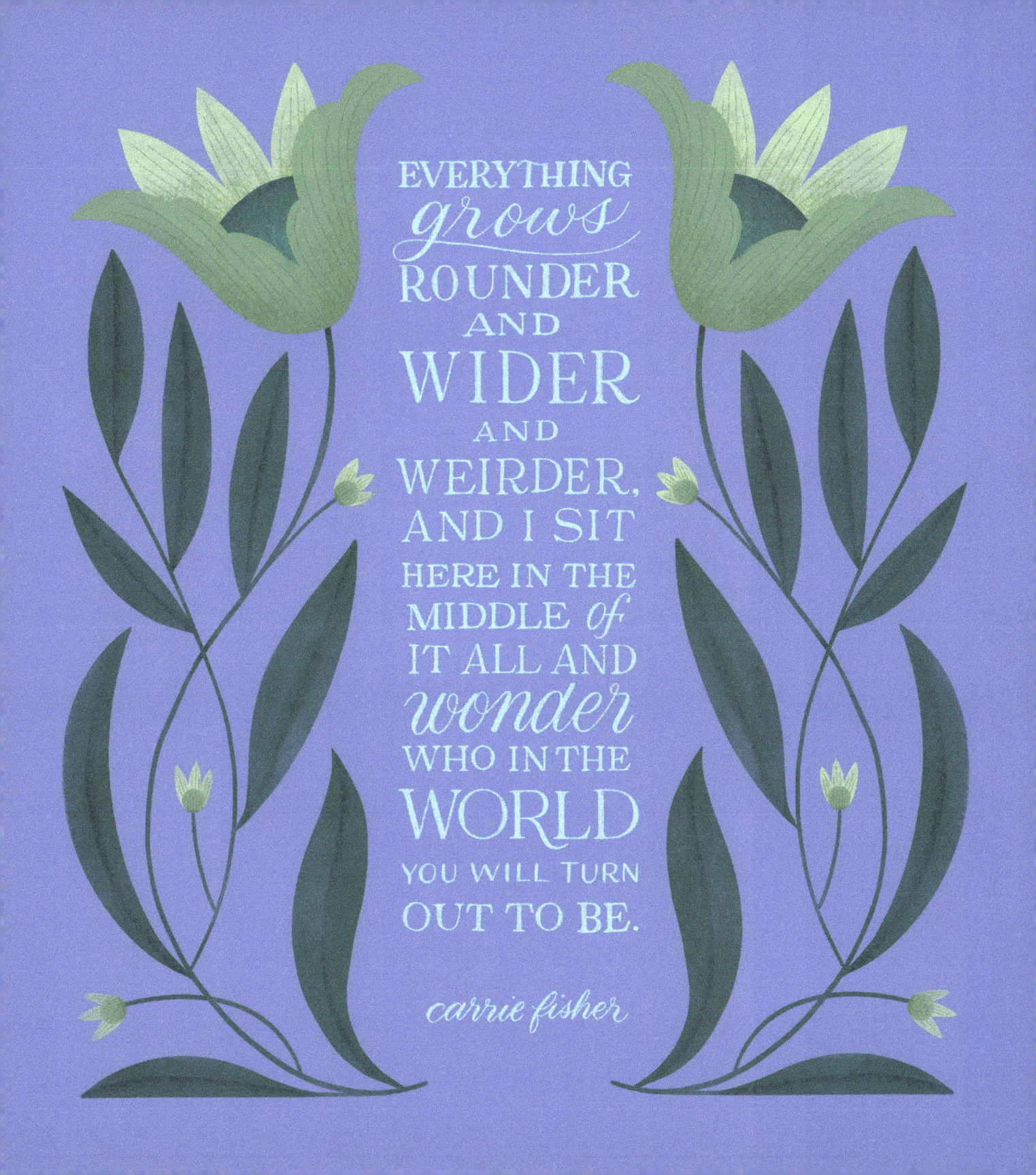

Everything *grows* rounder and wider and weirder, and I sit here in the middle *of* it all and *wonder* who in the world you will turn out to be.

carrie fisher

MONTH 8: FIRST-TIME MOM'S FIRSTS

First time you felt like you were waddling _____

First time you felt a contraction _____

First time the doctor/midwife checked you for dilation _____

First time someone asked, "You're still pregnant?" _____

First time you felt swelling and your shoes and/or jewelry didn't fit _____

WEEKS 29 TO 32

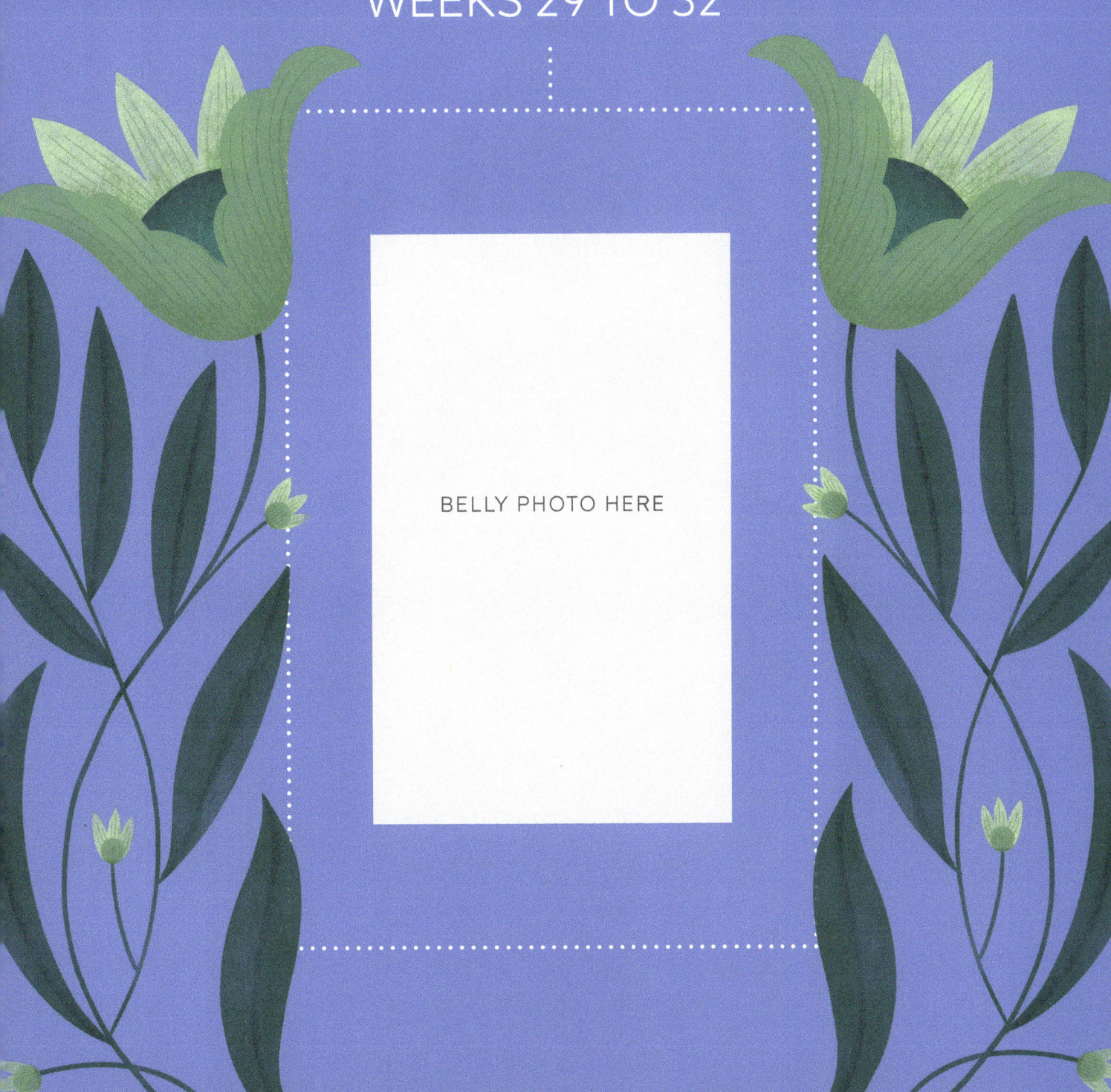

BELLY PHOTO HERE

SIZE COMPARISON

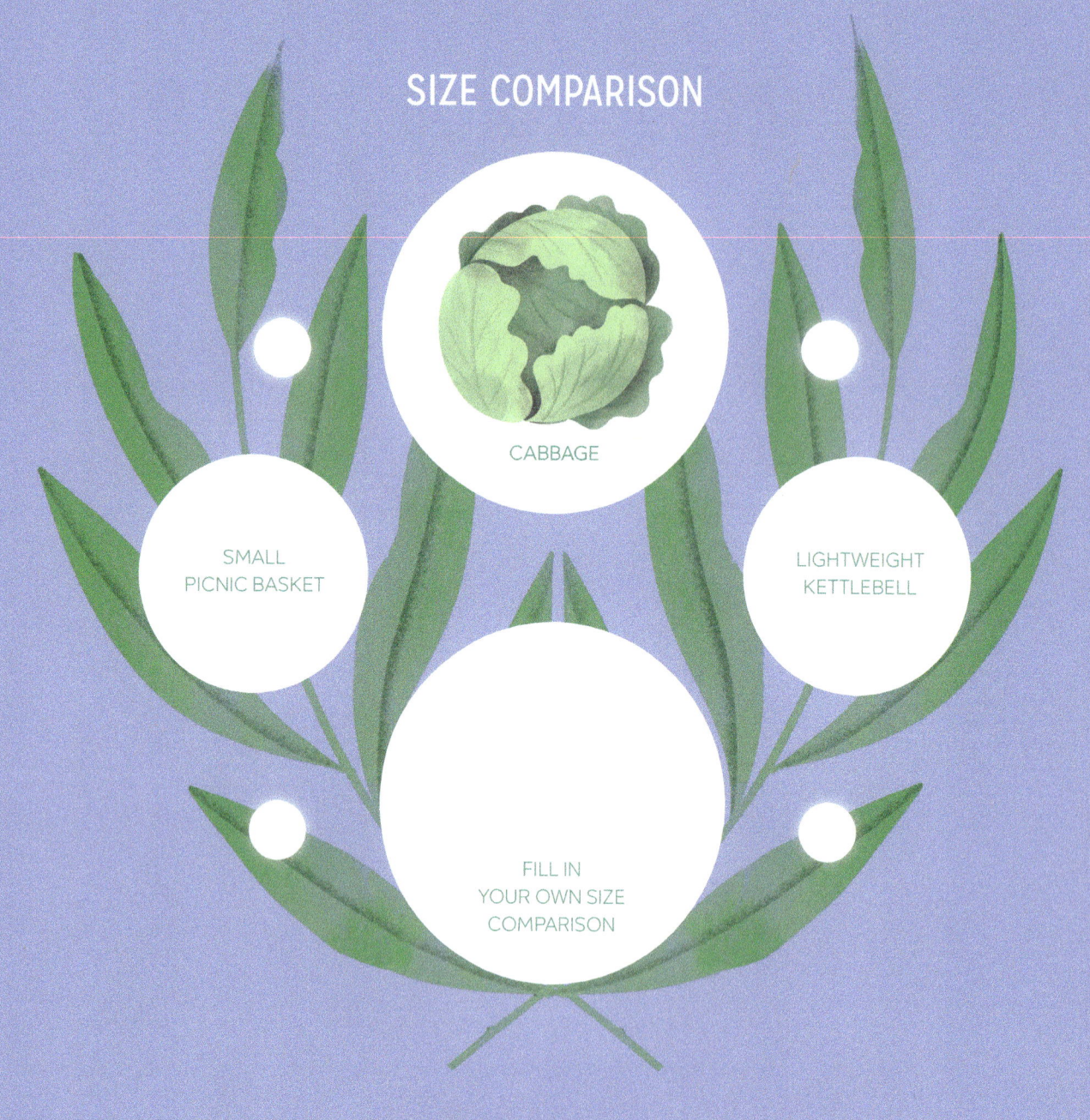

CABBAGE

SMALL PICNIC BASKET

LIGHTWEIGHT KETTLEBELL

FILL IN YOUR OWN SIZE COMPARISON

By the end of this month, your baby is about 17 inches long and weighs over 4 pounds.

PREGNANCY STATS TRACKER

Body

Have you felt more emotional lately? _____
_____

Have you felt anxious, nervous, or overwhelmed? _____
_____

Have you had any heartburn? _____
_____

Do you need to go to the bathroom quite frequently? _____
_____

Are you experiencing any hot flashes? _____
_____

How often have you felt regular or Braxton Hicks contractions? _____
_____

If your doctor/midwife has checked you for dilation, how dilated were you? ____
_____

Baby

Do you feel like your baby has dropped? _____

Is there any added pressure or tightness? _____

_____

Do you think your baby will come earlier or later than your due date? (Remember, only 5 percent of babies arrive on their actual due date.) _____

_____

PRENATAL APPOINTMENTS

DATE	WEEK	WEIGHT	TESTS CONDUCTED	QUESTIONS FOR DOCTOR/MIDWIFE

MONTH 8 CHECKLIST

Home

- Make any final changes you'd like in your home to prepare for the baby.
- If you had a baby shower, organize the gifts and purchase anything else you still need. (Remember, babies don't need a ton—just food, a safe place to sleep, and lots of lovin'.)
- _____
- _____
- _____

Self-Care

- Try not to overschedule so you can enjoy these last few weeks of pregnancy. You don't want to push yourself too hard.
- Do breathing exercises.
- Do Kegel exercises.
- Say personal affirmations or birth affirmations to yourself regularly.

- Get all your pampering done now. Once your baby is here, you won't feel like you have time. You deserve a good mani-pedi, haircut, and anything else that makes you feel good.
- _____
- _____
- _____

Baby

- Decide on a name for your baby.
- Count kicks and monitor movement closely.
- Watch for true labor contractions versus Braxton Hicks contractions, and start timing the distance between any contractions.
- _____
- _____
- _____

Medical

- Plan for hospital visitors. Do you want family and friends to come right after you give birth? Do you want to space out your visitors? If you have a preference, be sure to openly communicate your wishes to your family and friends, as well as to your doctor/midwife and the hospital.

- Watch for your mucus plug. (If you don't know what that plug looks like or what it is, feel free to Google it. It's another one of those "fun" pregnancy things.)
- _____
- _____
- _____

Important Events

- If you're documenting your delivery, make sure to be in contact with your photographer/videographer, so they know when to arrive and where to go.
- Create a group text that includes close friends and family so that your significant other or a family member can easily send updates when you leave for the hospital and during and after delivery.
- _____
- _____
- _____

DAILY REMINDERS

- Drink 10 cups of water over the course of the day.
- Take your prenatal vitamin.
- Eat at least three meals and three snacks.

Activity #1

Draw a funny picture of what you think your belly looks like.

Activity #2

During a contraction, circle the word "breathe" in the middle
of the page. Then relax your jaw. Focus on your breathing.
Close your eyes and repeat the strength word you chose in month 7.
Each time you feel a contraction, repeat these steps.

Breathe.

Activity #3

Draw a line from one dot to another that illustrates your moods throughout your pregnancy. For example, if you felt like you were level-headed, your line will be straight. If you experienced mood fluctuations, your line will fluctuate, too.

Activity #4

You've come a long way since you first found out you were pregnant. Create a list of 10 things that have helped you through this amazing transition.

1. _____
2. _____
3. _____
4. _____
5. _____
6. _____
7. _____
8. _____
9. _____
10. _____

Gratitude

What has given you the most joy this past month?

_____
_____
_____
_____
_____

Challenge

What part of the unknown—your delivery and life afterward—worries you the most?

_____
_____
_____
_____
_____

Reflection

Do you think motherhood will come naturally to you? Why or why not?

_____
_____
_____
_____
_____

Observation

Looking back over the past eight months, what has pregnancy been like for you? Has it been a breeze? Hard? Scary? Joyful? Painful? Describe your experience.

_____
_____
_____
_____
_____

FREESTYLE JOURNAL

Instead of wishing away nine months of pregnancy... I'd have cherished every moment and realized that the wonderment growing inside me was to be my only chance in life to assist God in a miracle.

— ERMA BOMBECK

MONTH 9: FIRST-TIME MOM'S FIRSTS

First consistent contractions _____

First sign of labor _____

First place you were when labor started _____

First person to help you with the delivery _____

WEEKS 33 TO 36

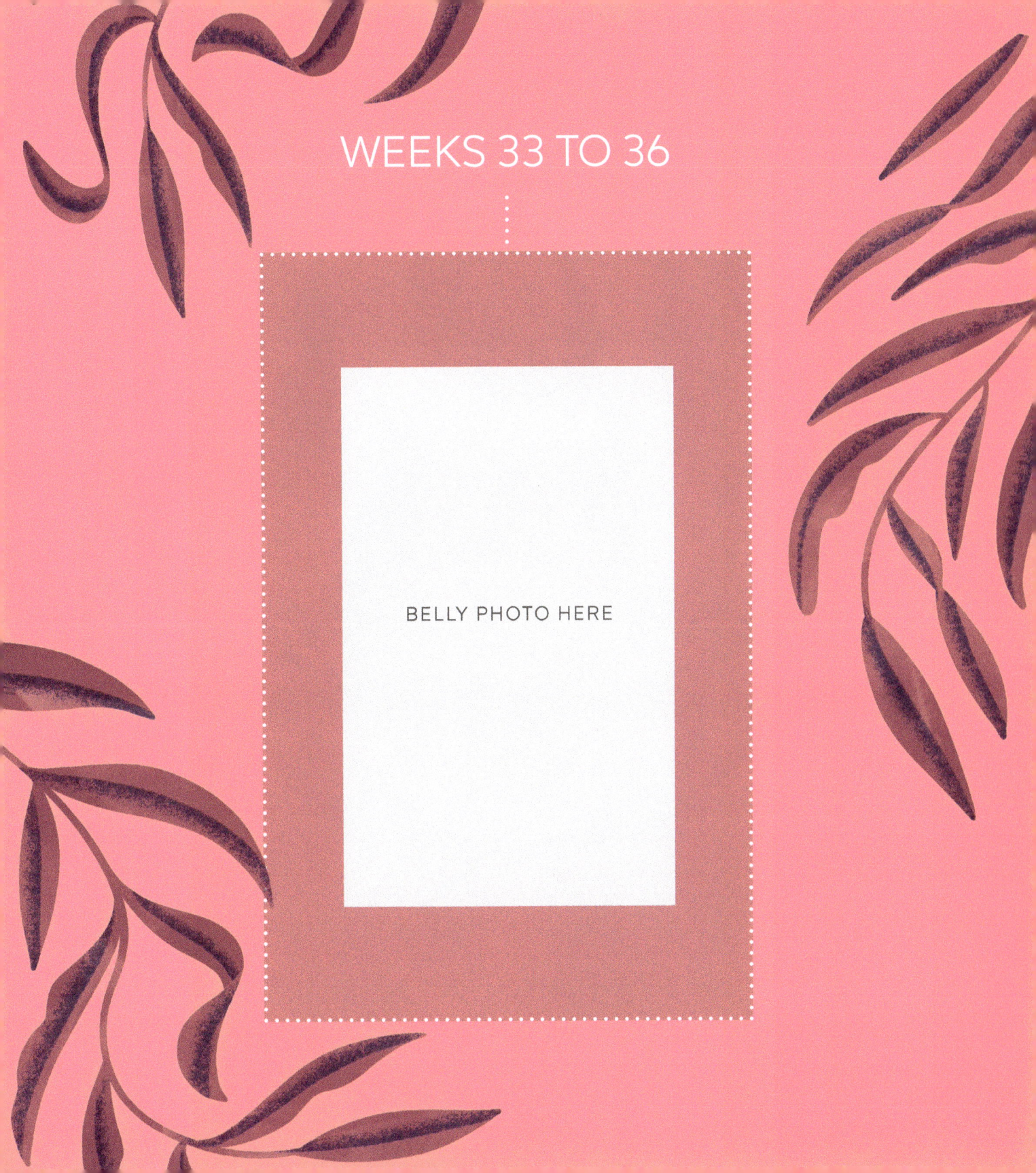

BELLY PHOTO HERE

SIZE COMPARISON

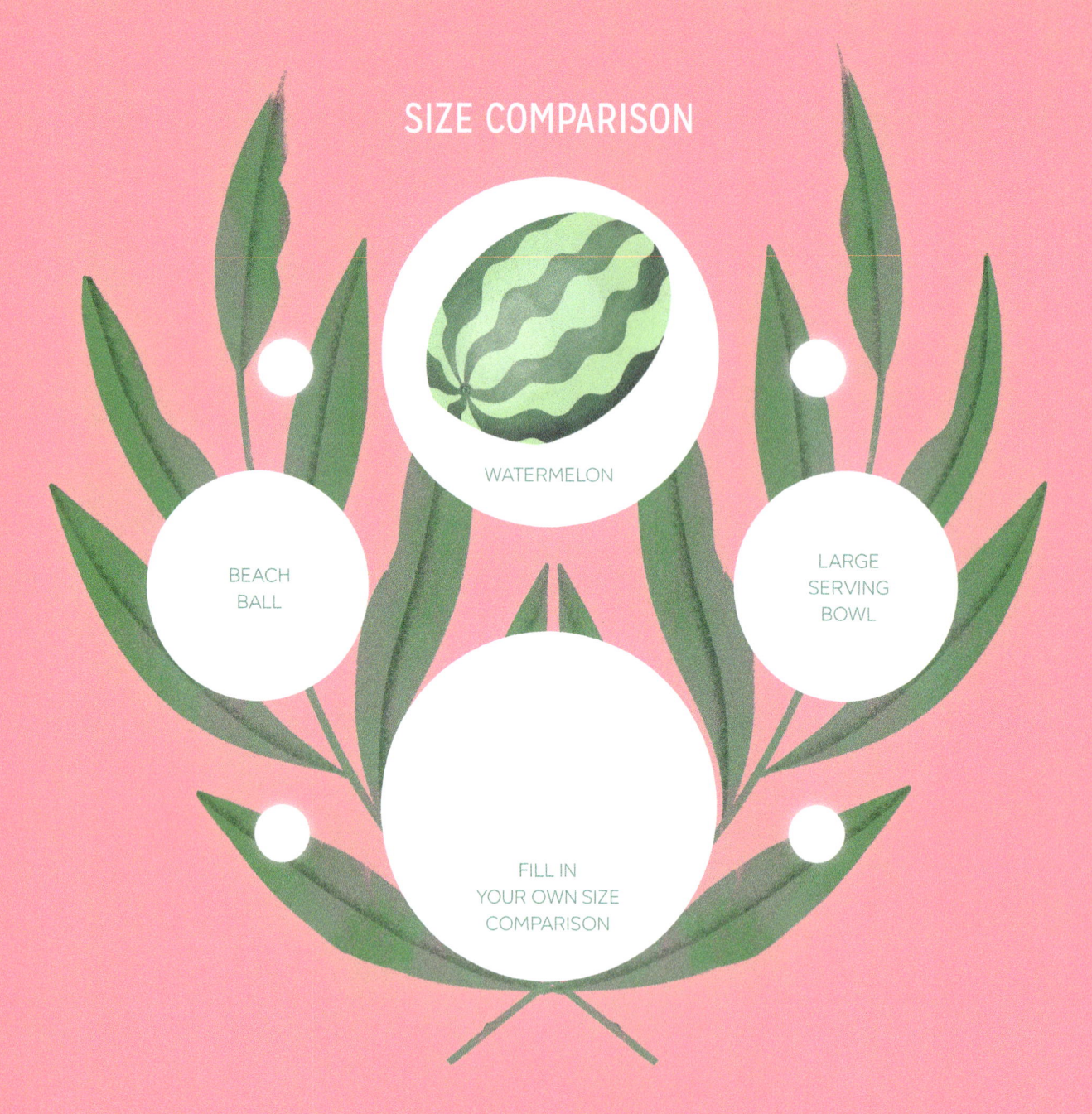

WATERMELON

BEACH BALL

LARGE SERVING BOWL

FILL IN YOUR OWN SIZE COMPARISON

By the end of this month, your baby is about 20 inches long and weighs about 7 pounds.

PREGNANCY STATS TRACKER

Body

Have you started labor? _____
_____

Are there any signs of your mucus plug? _____
_____

Has your water broken? _____
_____

How much are you dilated? _____
_____

Baby

Do you know the size of your baby? _____
_____

Which direction is your baby facing? _____
_____

Has your doctor/midwife expressed any concerns about delivery? _____
_____
_____
_____

PRENATAL APPOINTMENTS

DATE	WEEK	WEIGHT	TESTS CONDUCTED	QUESTIONS FOR DOCTOR/MIDWIFE

MONTH 9 CHECKLIST

Home

- Pack your hospital bag.
- Straighten up your house one last time before the baby comes home.
- Give an extra set of house keys to a family member so they can help bring things back and forth to the hospital if needed or in case you forget something.
- _____
- _____
- _____

Self-Care

- Rest as much as you can.
- Believe in yourself. You are made to give birth and be a mother.
- Meditate. This can be as simple as taking three deep breaths and thinking of three things you are grateful for. If you have fears or anxious feelings about labor and delivery, meditation can help.
- _____
- _____
- _____

Baby

- Keep counting those kicks and monitoring your baby's movement.
- Get nonstress tests if your doctor/midwife recommends them.
- _____
- _____
- _____

Medical

- Your doctor/midwife will tell you exactly when you need to get to the hospital. Make sure you are clear on what signs to look for, and go to the hospital as soon as you think you need to.
- Contact the hospital in advance and register for delivery.
- _____
- _____
- _____

Important Events

- If you have a planned delivery for whatever reason (such as a C-section or induction), make sure to get it scheduled.
- You're about to figure out the most important event of all: your baby's birthday!
- _____
- _____
- _____

DAILY REMINDERS

○	○	○
Drink 10 cups of water over the course of the day.	Take your prenatal vitamin.	Eat at least three meals and three snacks.

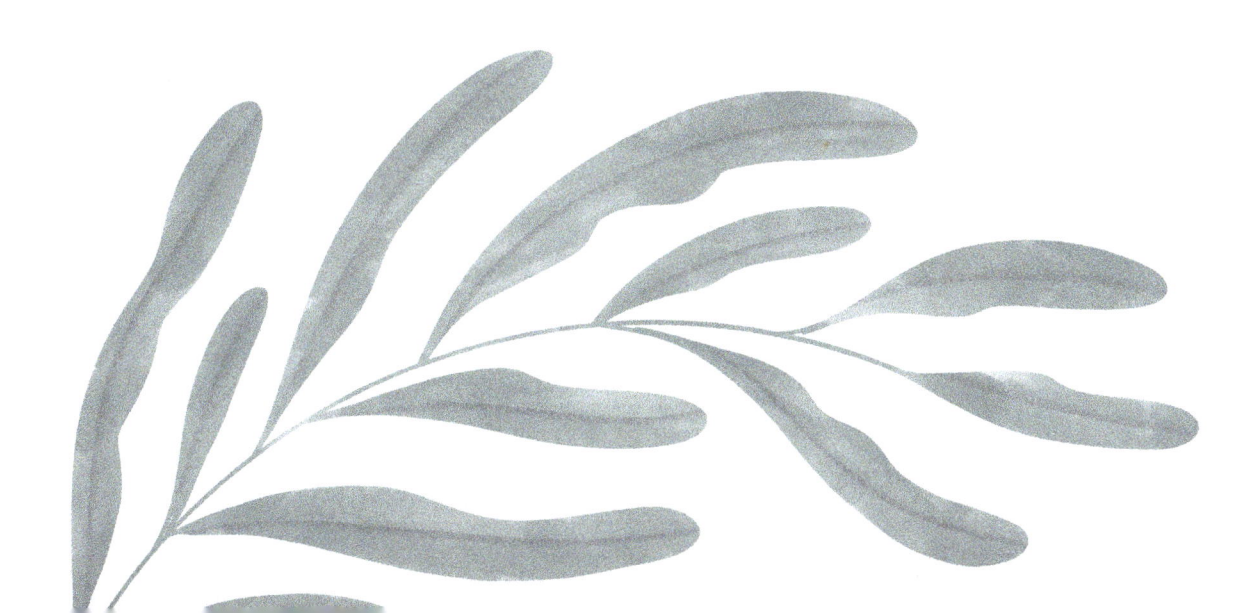

Activity #1

Make a list of all the things you will need help with after you give birth. Share the list with your significant other or a close friend and discuss anything that's not clear.

_____

_____

_____

_____

_____

_____

_____

_____

_____

_____

_____

Activity #2

Write your baby's name in the middle of the page in bubble letters and color it in.

Activity #3

Inside the heart, write all the positive feelings you are having right now. If you have negative feelings—which is perfectly fine—write them outside the heart. But try to focus on the feelings inside the heart.

Activity #4

Take a moment to allow any negativity you may be feeling to drain out of your body. Reflect on how strong your body is. Write down all the positive words you can think of with regard to your body. It has taken you through almost nine months of pregnancy, and that is amazing!

_____

_____

_____

_____

_____

_____

_____

_____

_____

_____

Gratitude

What are your feelings toward your baby now that it is almost time to meet this little person?

_____
_____
_____
_____
_____

Challenge

What were your most pressing difficulties this month?

_____
_____
_____
_____
_____

Reflection

What do you look forward to the most about the delivery? What aren't you looking forward to?

_____
_____
_____
_____
_____

Observation

What have been your favorite and least favorite parts of your pregnancy?

_____
_____
_____
_____
_____

FREESTYLE JOURNAL

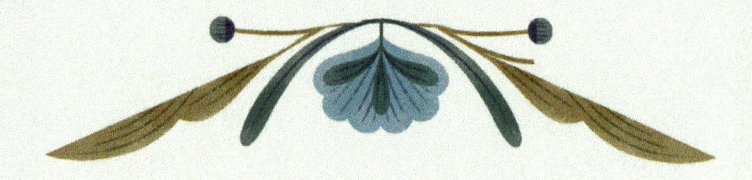

You're Here!

GENDER	
TIME BORN	
PLACE	
WEIGHT	
LENGTH	

Hello, Baby!

NEWBORN PHOTO HERE

About the Author

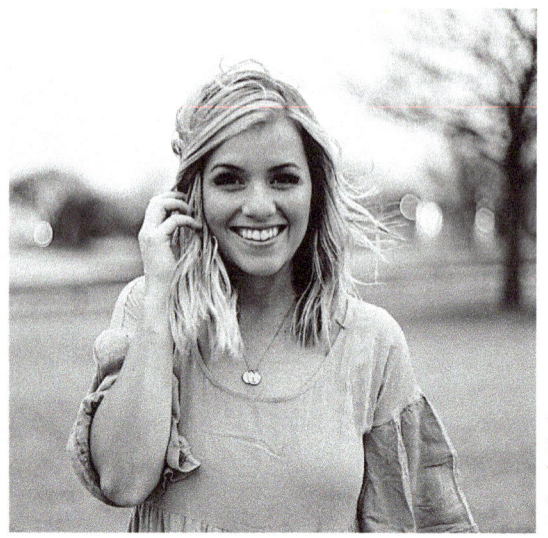

© Sarah Clark

Aubrey Grossen is a wife and mama to three kids. After having her first baby, she suffered through postpartum depression. As a result, she created an online community. It started off with just under 40 close friends and family members, and over the years, it has grown to tens of thousands of moms. Writing is her outlet, and she has grown her blogging business since 2014. She blogs regularly on the Mamahood Blog (themamahoodblog.com), has joined forces with another mama in launching a podcast (The Mamahood Podcast), and loves hosting events as well.

Motherhood wasn't something that came naturally for her, but it has been one of the greatest blessings in her life. She fought through a rough patch of pregnancies and miscarriages to get her babies here. She finds joy in traveling with her family, spending time with her kids and husband, and having a bowl of late-night ice cream in bed while watching her favorite shows.

CPSIA information can be obtained
at www.ICGtesting.com
Printed in the USA
BVHW051629140120
569265BV00003B/6

9 781641 524506